CLINICAL USE OF ANTIBODIES

Developments in Nuclear Medicine

VOLUME 19

Series Editor: Peter H. Cox

The titles published in this series are listed at the end of this volume.

Clinical Use of Antibodies

Tumours, infection, infarction, rejection and in the diagnosis of AIDS

edited by

RICHARD P. BAUM
Department of Nuclear Medicine,
University Medical Center, Frankfurt, Germany

PETER H. COX
Department of Nuclear Medicine,
Daniel den Hoed Clinic, Rotterdam, The Netherlands

GUSTAV HÖR
Department of Nuclear Medicine,
University Medical Center, Frankfurt, Germany

and

GIAN LUIGI BURAGGI
Division of Nuclear Medicine,
National Tumour Institute, Milan, Italy

SPRINGER-SCIENCE+BUSINESS MEDIA, B.V.

Library of Congress Cataloging-in-Publication Data

Clinical use of antibodies : tumours, infection, infarction, rejection, and in the diagnosis of AIDS / edited by Richard P. Baum ... [et al.].
p. cm. -- (Developments in nuclear medicine ; v. 19)
Based on lectures held at an international symposium organized as a post congress meeting of the German Nuclear Medicine Congress which took place in Frankfurt/Main in March 1990, under the auspices of the Task Group Cardiology and the Task Group on Clinical Utility of Labelled Antibodies of the European Association of Nuclear Medicine.
Includes index.
ISBN 978-94-010-5555-0 ISBN 978-94-011-3516-0 (eBook)
DOI 10.1007/978-94-011-3516-0
1. Radioimmunoimaging--Congresses. 2. Radioimmunotherapy--Congresses. 3. Monoclonal antibodies--Congresses. I. Baum, Richard P., 1954- . II. European Association of Nuclear Medicine. Task Group Cardiology. III. European Association of Nuclear Medicine. Task Group on Clinical Utility of Labelled Antibodies. IV. Deutschen Gesellschaft für Nuklearmedizin. Kongress (1990 : Frankfurt am Main, Germany) V. Series: Developments in nuclear medicine ; 19.
[DNLM: 1. Antibodies--therapeutic use--congresses. W1 DE998KF v. 19 / QW 575 C6416 1990]
RC78.7.R38C48 1991
616.07'57--dc20
DNLM/DLC
for Library of Congress 91-20881

ISBN 978-94-010-5555-0

Printed on acid-free paper

Contents

Preface

It was at Frankfurt/Main in 1899 that Paul Ehrlich first expounded his famous "site-chain theory" - which described the basic immunological principal of antibody-antigen interaction - on the occasion of the opening of the Institute for Experimental Therapeutics (which was later named after him). Nearly 100 years have passed since, and in retrospect it can be said that the "Ehrlich Era" (first steps in immunology "Magic Bullet" concept) and the "Behring Era" (detection of antibodies and serum therapy) formed the essential basis in the development of immunology. Niels K.Jerne, the former director of the Paul Ehrlich Institute in Frankfurt/Main received, together with Georges Köhler and Cesar Milstein, the Nobel Prize in Medicine 1984. These late successors of Ehrlich and Behring first described the hybridoma technology (in 1975) which enabled one of the most important and revolutionary technological innovations in the field of immunology - the production of monoclonal antibodies.

It happens that, the time of the publication of this book, just a decade has passed since the first use of radiolabelled monoclonal antibodies in man (by the Lausanne Group). Over these 10 years a tremendous progress has taken place in the field of immunoscintigraphy: A large panel of highly specific monoclonal antibodies against tumour-associated antigens as well as normal cell compounds have been developed. Enormous progress has been made in the field of radiolabelling - from iodine-131 to technetium-99m or even positron-emitting radionuclides, e.g. iodine-124. More and more clinical applications are studied, not only in the field of oncology, but also for the detection of non-malignant conditions.

This book is intended to present a current perspective of the clinical use of antibodies. It is derived from the lectures held at the International Symposium (organised as a Post Congress Meeting of the German Nuclear Medicine Congress which took place in Frankfurt/Main in March 1990) under the auspices of the Task Group Cardiology (Chairman: Prof.Dr.G.Hör, Frankfurt/Main) and the Task Group on Clinical Utility of Labelled Antibodies (Chairman: Prof.Dr. G.L. Buraggi, Milano) of the European Association of Nuclear Medicine.

The contributing authors are leading experts in their respective fields and I am grateful that they enabled the rapid production of these proceedings. This would not have been possible, however, with the great help of Prof.Dr.Peter Cox, Rotterdam, who spent considerable effort in revising, correcting and proof-reading the manuscripts.

Richard P.Baum

Frankfurt/Main, March 1991

List of Contributors

A. Bamias
ICRF Oncology Group
RPMS
Hammersmith Hospital
Ducane Road
LONDON W12 0NN
U.K.

Co-authors: J.M. Sackier, H.P. Kalofonos, B. Dhokia, D. Snook, K. Bosslet, C. Wood and A.A. Epenetos

R.P. Baum
Department of Nuclear Medicine
University Medical Center
Theodor-Stern-Kai 7
DW-6000 FRANKFURT/Main 70
Germany

S. Bhattacharya
Northwick Park Hospital
and Clinical Research Centre
Watford Road
HARROW, Middlesex HA1 3UJ
U.K.

Co-author: A. Lahiri

K. Bosslet
Research Laboratories of Behringwerke AG
P.O. Box 1140
DW-3550 MARBURG/Lahn
Germany

Co-authors: A. Steinstraesser, P. Hermentin, L. Kuhlmann, A. Bruynck, M. Magerstaedt, G. Seemann, A. Schwarz and H.H. Sedlacek

G.L. Buraggi
Nuclear Medicine Division
Instituto Nazionale Tumori
Via Venezian 1
20133 MILAN
Italy

I. Carrio
Nuclear Medicine Unit
Hospital de Sant Pau
Avda San Antonio Maria Claret 167
08025 BARCELONA
Spain

J.F. Chatal
Centre René Gauducheau
and University Hospital
Unite 211, INSERM
F-44035 NANTES Cedex
France

Co-authors: A. Chetanneau, P. Peltier, C. Curtet and P.A. Lehur

P.H. Cox
Department of Nuclear Medicine
Daniel den Hoed Clinic
P.O. Box 5201
3008 AE ROTTERDAM

Co-author: K. Kristensen

D.M. Goldenberg
Centre for Molecular Medicine
and Immunology
1 Bruce Street
NEWARK, NJ 07103
U.S.A.

M. Granowska
Department of Nuclear Medicine
St. Bartholomew's Hospital
West Smithfield
LONDON EC1A 7BE
U.K.

Co-authors: K.E. Britton, S.J. Mather, M. Naeem, T. Jobling and J.H. Sheperd

G. Hör
Department of Nuclear Medicine
University Medical Center
Theodor-Stern-Kai 7
DW-6000 FRANKFURT/Main 70
Germany

M. Mali
The Department of Nuclear Medicine
Montefiore Medical Center
Albert Einstein College of Medicine
BRONX, NY 10461
U.S.A.

Co-author: L.M. Freeman

D.L. Munz
Department of Nuclear Medicine
Georg August University Gottingen
Robert Koch Str 40
DW-3400 GOTTINGEN
Germany

Co-authors: D. Sandrock, A.J. Morguet and A. Enderle

A.A. Noujaim
Biomira Inc.
9411 20th Avenue
EDMONTON, Alberta
Canada T6N 1E5

Co-authors: T.R. Sykes, A.J. McEwan, G.D. McClean, S.A. McQuarrie, G. Stanczyk and B.M. Longnecker

A.C. Perkins
Department of Medical Physics
and Vascular Surgery
Queens Medical Center
NOTTINGHAM NG7 2UH
U.K.

Co-author: R.J. Lonsdale

G.V. Wangenheim
Paul-Ehrlich Institute
Paul-Ehrlich Str 51-59
DW-6070 LANGEN/Hessen
Germany

Co-author: J. Lower

ADVANCES IN CANCER IMAGING AND THERAPY WITH RADIOLABELLED ANTIBODIES

D.M. Goldenberg

Monoclonal antibody (MAb) technology has generated considerable interest in the development of approaches to improve the management of cancer patients, as well as our understanding of some aspects of the malignant process (1-3). A very large number of rodent MAbs have been developed for the use in the diagnosis, detection, monitoring, and treatment of various neoplasms, many of which have been generated against tumor-associated antigens, growth factor receptors and other molecules. In diagnosis and detection, these MAbs have been used to quantitate and monitor circulating tumor markers, identify markers of cell types and certain pathological changes in tissue specimens, and to detect sites of cancer by external imaging methods (2). Therapeutically they have been used either as unconjugated ("naked") antibodies or to target drugs, toxins, effector lymphocytes, cytokines, and radionuclides to tumors (3-5).

Although the overall results of using naked MAb therapy (involving rodent MAbs) have been disappointing, these efforts have contributed to our knowledge of how such reagents can exert antitumor effects. Three principle mechanisms include (1) inhibition of cell growth by direct binding to cell surfaces, (2) cooperation with host effector mechanisms to lyse tumor cells coated with antibody, and (3) alteration of the host's immune system to initiate tumor rejection. The obstacles that have faced the use of unconjugated MAbs appear to also hinder drug, toxin, and radionuclide immunoconjugate therapy; namely, (1) the presence of circulating free antigen which can complex the injected MAb, (2) modulation or disappearance of the target antigen from the tumor cell, (3) heterogeneity of antigen expression, (4) low targeting and uptake of the injected MAb in the tumor(s) and (5) the immunogenicity of murine MAbs, resulting in human anti-mouse antibodies (HAMA). Another important consideration is the nature of the anticancer antibody. MAb technology has not resulted in reagents that are more specific for cancer than those identified with traditional polyclonal antibody methods. Most anticancer MAbs are relatively specific, reacting with malignant cells to a higher percentage than normal cells. Also, it is rare to find a MAb that is restricted even to a single cell type. They are usually reactive with many tumor types within a system, and more frequently are reactive with many

R. P. Baum et al. (eds.), Clinical Use of Antibodies, 1–13.

different cell types, as pan-carcinoma antibodies. The best known pan-carcinoma antibodies are against carcinoembryonic antigen (CEA), which react with carcinomas of many different organs and systems (6).

Radioimmunodetection (RAID)

Given these problems, it is no wonder that the first efforts to image cancers with radiolabelled antibodies, a process I called radioimmunodetection (or RAID) 12 years ago (7,8), were received with much skepticism (9). It was believed that the injected antibody, when made against a circulating cancer marker, such as CEA, would complex with CEA in the blood and thus never reach the tumor in adequate amounts for successful external scintigraphy (10.11). However, as frequently occurs in a new clinical endeavor, the predictions were untrue, and although complexes between CEA and anti-CEA antibodies were formed (12), these did not preclude tumor targeting and imaging with a radiolabelled antibody (8,13,14). In contrast, the major difficulty proved to be blood-pool and interstitial radioactivity due to a high retention of the radiolabelled 160-kD whole IgG in these compartments in the first few days after injection. In order to disclose sites of targeted radioactivity in the first 2 days, we had to rely on computer-assisted subtraction methods that compensated for blood-pool and interstitial non-specific radioactivity, and this resulted in high sensitivity of tumor imaging with different antibodies and different tumor types (8,14,15). However, this process required considerable skill and experience, since use of two different radionuclides (one on the MAb and the other as the subtraction agent) resulted in different pharmacokinetics and potential artifacts. Nevertheless, this early work proved the feasibility of RAID, and even showed that tumours missed by other radiological methods could be disclosed by RAID, thus indicating clinical utility (14,16). The early work was with purified polyclonal antibodies, so it was expected that MABs would, by themselves, improve RAID. This has not proven to be true, since problems of background radioactivity are still present with radiolabelled MAbs. But the wider availability of MAbs has resulted in a more widespread participation and, in turn, development of this technology (17). Antibodies and antibody forms have been improved, radionuclides with better imaging properties are now conjugated by simpler methods to the antibodies, and advanced imaging instruments and methods are more widespread (18,19). These advances and their impacts on RAID will be summarized.

Targeting Antibodies

Since the first use of purified polyclonal antibodies against CEA (8), a diverse array of murine MAbs against a number of tumour-associated antigens have entered clinical trials as imaging agents (Table 1). For the most part, these have been used a whole IgG preparations, and studies of HAMA responses in patients receiving only one injection of these preparations indicate that about 20-30 per cent show this immune reaction (20). It has also been found that antibody fragments, both the F(ab')2 and Fab' or Fab show more repaid tumour targeting as well as clearance from background tissues, thus permitting earlier imaging than with whole IgG (21-23). Further, the fragments, devoid of the more immunogenic Fc portion, how a lower frequency of HAMA responses, especially the monovalent Fab form (24). Antibody fragments, therefore, appear to be the preferred imaging agents, and efforts are now underway to assess whether even smaller fragment forms, such as single-chain antibodies, show even more desirable imaging properties.

Table 1. Cancers Targeted Clinically with Radiolabeled Antibodies

Cancer Type	Abs	Cancer Type	Abs
Colorectal	CEA 17-1A 19-9 791T/36 CSAp (MU-9) B72.3	Ovarian	CEA HMFG-2 791T/36 SM3 OC-125 OV-TL3 B72.3
Prostate	PAP PSA	Lymphomas	Ferritin Lym-1 Immu-LL2 T-101 MB-1
Melanoma	p97 96.5 9.2.27 225.28S ZME 018	Breast	CEA B72.3 HMFG MA-5
Lung	CEA NR-LU-10	Liver	AFP Ferritin
Trophoblast & Germ Cell	AFP HCG	Neuroblastoma	3F8 BW575/9

Since Fab forms have a high kidney uptake, thus making tumour imaging difficult in the immediate area of this organ (23), recent experimental results indicating that single-chain antibodies show rapid tumour targeting without renal accretion suggest that these may be yet another step toward an ideal antibody form for imaging, particularly for repeated use (25). With regard to the selection of an antibody for clinical use, there is little comparative evidence for those listed in Table 1. Although different groups report different results between these antibodies, this variation is undoubtedly due to different radionuclides, patient selection, interpretation criteria, etc., so it is very difficult to rank these MAbs as targeting agents in any specific tumour type. However, it appears that the most widely studied antibody has been that to CEA, and relatively high rates of detecting both known and occult tumours, particularly colorectal neoplasms, have been reported (14,16,21-23,28). The lower rates of sensitivity for the B72.3 MAb may be due to the more extensive use of 111-In as the label (discussed below) and the whole IgG form (29).

Radionuclides

The majority of studies in RAID during the first 5-7 years after the initial clinical reports involved 131-I as the label, because of its ready availability and the ease of labelling antibodies with this isotope. However, its relatively poor imaging properties and its beta-emission component make this less ideal than other radionuclides, such as 123-I, 111-In, and 99m-Tc. Studies with 124-I labelled CEA MAb fragments showed excellent imaging results (21-23). but the poor availability of this radionuclide (and the high cost) make it impractical. 111-In has been a favourite of many groups, showing excellent imaging characteristics, a favourable 2.6-day half-life, and generally easy and reproducible chelation-labelling methods. Its major limitation, however, has been a high retention in normal liver, thus making it difficult to disclose hot tumour sites in the liver for at least 2-3 days after injection of the preparation (30,31), thus affecting the accuracy of tumour detection in this prominent organ for tumour metastasis. The major problem with the use of 99m-Tc, as we encountered in 1980 (32), has been an inadequate binding to the antibody by direct or indirect (chelation) methods. It was also thought that this isotope's half life of 6-hr would be too short for adequate antibody targeting (21,33). Recent advances in direct labelling methods for attaching 99m-Tc to both whole IgG and Fab' fragments have resulted in very simple and convenient kits (34,35), so that the nuclear medicine department can now use generator-produced99m-Tc, at a very low cost, with simple, on site labelling kits. Clinical results with both 99m-Tc whole IgG or Fab' against CEA have shown very good colorectal cancer detection rates at about 24 hr for the whole IgG and 4 hr for the Fab' (23,27,36). It appears that the Fab' may be more suitable for tumour imaging in the liver at a few hours after injection than the whole IgG preparation (37), and that the Fab' kit may show less nonspecific intestinal activity than the whole IgG kit. However, the Fab' preparation shows considerably more renal activity than the whole IgG reagent, thus making interpretation of images in close proximity to this organ difficult, unless emission tomography is performed (36).

Imaging procedures

Early studies with RAID were restricted to planar imaging, and showed the capability of disclosing lesions in the size range of about 1.5 - 2.0 cm (13,16). Single-photon emission computed tomography, or SPECT, later showed that smaller tumours could be disclosed with 111-In or 99m-Tc-labelled antibodies, even lesions as small as 0.5 cm or less (23,26,36). However, SPECT requires considerably longer imaging sessions as well as more user expertise than when planar scanning is done.

Taking all of these factors into consideration, it appears that from the vantage point of safety (low immunogenicity), rapidity (earliest imaging sessions), labelling ease and efficacy (sensitivity and disclosure of occult lesions), 99m-Tc labelled antibody fragments are the currently available ideal imaging agents. This should now be tested by comparing the same antibody as a whole IgG or fragment labelled with 111-In or 99m-Tc in the same or a similar group of patients. Our own initial comparison of 99m-Tc-labelled IgG and Fab' CEA MAbs in the same patients have indicated an advantage for the Fab' preparation at the 4 hr imaging session in the disclosure of liver metastasis (37). Also, since single injections of the Fab' have not resulted in any elevations of HAMA to date, whereas 20-30 percent of patients receiving intact IGG show abnormal GAMA responses, the Fab' form appears to be a safer preparation.

Radioimmunotherapy (RAIT)

Advances in clinical cancer RAIT have not been as successful as those in RAID, particularly in the therapy of solid tumours. Bone marrow toxicity, with major effects on the leukocytes and thrombocytes, has been observed as the dose-limiting toxicity (38,39). One of the main factors responsible for the modest clinical effects achieved to date is the low tumour accretion of antibodies (usually 0,01 to 0,001 percent of the injected dose per gram of tumour) (40,41), which limits the cGy dose delivered to tumour. In RAID, only a differential ratio of counts in tumour as compared to adjacent tissues is required for successful imaging, whereas RAIT depends on dose and duration of radioactivity delivered relatively selectively to the tumour. The majority of studies have involved 131-I conjugated to murine whole IgG antibodies, and at present there is a paucity of evidence that radioiodinated MAbs by themselves have shown consistent and reproducible, major responses in solid cancers. Order and his colleagues at the Johns Hopkin's Cancer Centre have demonstrated that when combined with other therapy modalities, anti-ferritin antibodies made in different animals and conjugated with 131-I can have important response rates of 40 percent in hepatocellular cancer (42). Even better results with radioiodinated antibodies alone have been reported in patients with radiosensitive lymphatic tumours, such as Hodgkin's disease (43) and T- and B-cell lymphomas (44-47) In the lymphoma patients, moreover, there appears to be a low frequency of HAMA induced, which is probably related to the immunosuppressed nature of the lymphoma patients (48). These encouraging findings support the view that RAIT, if it can overcome the relatively low radiation doses now delivered to tumours, could eventually play an important role in cancer therapy. Unfortunately, the tumour doses achieved to date usually have been less than 2,000 cGy. In hepatocellular carcinoma, Order et al. reported tumour doses of 1,100 - 1,200 cGy on the average, resulting in therapeutic responses when combined with doxorubicin and fluorouracil (42). Although the cGy doses delivered to lymphomas have been in this range or less, they appear to be preferred targets for RAIT because of their radiosensitivity, their good vascularization, and as already mentioned, their patients having a poorer or infrequent HAMA response. Our own recent studies with a new B-cell specific antibody, EPB-2 (or LL2) (49), have demonstrated very good targeting in non-Hodgkin's B-cell lymphoma, as well as responses to low doses (6.2-50.0 mCi; 0.2-3.9 mg) of 131-I-labelled MAb (47). These encouraging results with this B-cell lymphoma MAb have stimulated our expansion of these studies to evaluate the effects of higher doses of radioactivity and of antibody.

Although 131-I has dominated cancer RAIT, interest has been generated by 125-I, 90-Y, 67-Cu, 186-Re, 188-Re, 212-Bi, and 211-At. 125-I emits Auger electrons, whose short-range energy can effect the nucleus and thus destroy cells once the electrons are internalized. This isotope is being used in conjugation with MAbs against epidermal growth factor receptor in patients with glioma. 90-Y is a pure beta emitter of 0.937 meV with a physical half-life of 2.7 days, and appears to permit the delivery of higher radiation doses to tumour than 131-I-MAbs, but probably at increased host toxicity. One of the problems with this metallic radionuclide is the difficulty in achieving a tight and stable linkage to MAb, resulting in bone toxicity (50). However, improved chelates that may reduce or avoid this problem are in development and evaluation (51,52). 67-Cu is also being studied by chelation linkage to MAbs, particularly in lymphoma therapy (53). 186-Re and 188-Re have gained interest recently because of the similarity in their chemical properties to 99m-Tc (54) 186-Re has an average beta energy of 0.781 meV and a physical half-life of 3.8 days, while 188-Re has a maximum beta energy of 2.116 meV and a physical half-life of 17 hr. Both have the additional advantage, in contrast to 90-Y, of having a gamma energy component which can be used for imaging and quantitation of uptake. In addition to the beta-emitting isotopes, alpha emission from 212-Bi and 211-At, which irradiate at very short distances, have been used in laboratory studies (55,56) and appear to be promising radionuclides for the therapy of micrometastases, circulating tumour cells, or small nodules.

It is apparent that many potential therapeutic radionuclides for conjugation to MAbs are available, but the major problem has been achieving tight and stable linkage by simple methods, without affecting the MAb's immunoreactivity and targeting properties. As advances in bioconjugate radiochemistry are made, more of these radionuclide-MAb combinations will enter clinical RAIT trials. However, methods to increase the radiation doses delivered to tumour, as well as to reduce or avoid the induction of a response to the foreign immunoglobulin, need to be developed. The particular advantage of RAIT over other forms of immunoconjugate therapy is that the radiation deposited by an antibody can destroy cells at a distance, thus not requiring antibody uptake by each tumour cell. Depending on the form of radiation, the distance can be large, as with beta emitters, or short, as with alpha energy and Auger electrons. Thus, beta emitters may be more appropriate for large tumours, and those isotopes emitting energy traversing short distances are better suited for the treatment of very small tumours or disseminated cells.

The administration of high and repeated doses of radiolabelled MAbs has been limited by the HAMA response and by myelotoxicity. The former may be avoided by the development and use of human or humanized MAbs (57,58), while the latter may be overcome by autologous bone marrow transplantation (46) and/or the administration of marrow-stimulating cytokines, such as IL-1, IL-3, G-CSF, GM-CSF, etc. In an experimental model system, we have shown the potential advantage of combining IL-1 with RAIT (59), and this is now being expanded to Gm-CSF (60).

Cancer RAIT is currently a very active area of research, with studies involving the selection of antibody and antibody form, radionuclide and conjugation chemistry, methods to enhance MAb accretion in tumour and decrease marrow toxicity. It also is apparent that RAIT may find its role in cancer therapy either as an adjuvant to surgery, where disseminated cells and occult tumour can be irradiated, or in combination with chemotherapy to remit advanced malignancy. These prospects will require sophisticated animal and clinical studies, once the basic issues of radiobiology, bioconjugate chemistry, antigen site, quantity and expression, antibody form, structure and immunogenicity and tumour accretion of the therapeutic agent, are elucidated.

Conclusion

Monoclonal antibodies made against a variety of cancer-associated antigens have been labelled with gamma-emitting radionuclides, such as 99m-Tc, and used in vivo for cancer imaging. This approach has complemented other radiological methods, such as computed tomography, and revealed occult lesions in various sites, thus contributing to patient management. The conjugation of therapeutic radionuclides (Auger electrons, beta and alpha-emitters) has resulted in experimental and clinical evidence of cancer radioimmunotherapy. RAIT has proved to be a more difficult endeavour than cancer radioimmunodetection. At present, the best clinical results of radioimmunotherapy have been observed in patients with radiosensitive lymphatic neoplasms, even at very low doses of radiation and MAb. Advances in antibody specificity, radionuclide conjugation, antibody re-engineering to reduce immunogenicity, antibody uptake, and the reduction of myelotoxicity should increase the potential of cancer radioimmunotherapy.

Acknowledgements

I thank Robert M.Sharkey, Ph.D., Jo Ann Horowitz, M.D., Thomas C.Hall, M.D.,Robert E.Lee, Karen A. Burger,M.D., Sumathi Murthy, M.D., Lawrence C.Swayne, M.D., Edith

Higginbotham-Ford, M.D., Jeffry Siegel, Ph.D., Rosalyn D. Blumenthal, Ph.D., Hildegard Goldenberg, M.D., Daniel O. Izon, M.D., Hans J.Hansen Ph.D., and Carl M.Pinsky,M.D., for their participation in our radioimmunodetectionand radioimmunotherapyprograms.

This work has been supported in part by USPHS grant CA39841 from the NIH, by the New Jersey Commission on Science and Technology, and by the New Jersey State Commission on Cancer Research.

References

1.Sell S. and Reisfeld R.A.(eds.)[1985] Monoclonal Antibodies in Cancer, Humana Press. Clifton.N.J.pp.1-428.

2.Schlom J.[1986] Basic principles and application of monoclonal antibodies in the management of carcinomas: The Richard and Hinda Rosenthal Foundation award lecture, Cancer Res. 45: 3225-3238.

3.Foon K.A.[1989] Biological response modifiers: the new immunotherapy, Cancer Res. 49, 1621-1639.

4.Vogel C.W. (ed.)[1987] Immunoconjugates. Antibody Conjugates in Radioimmunoimaging and Therapy of Cancer, Oxford University Press. N.Y.pp3-308.

5.Harris D.T. and Mastrangelo M.J.[1989] Serotherapy of cancer, Semin Oncol. 16. 180-198.

6.Goldenberg D.M. et al.[1976] Carcinoembryonic antigen in histopathology: immunoperoxidasestaining of conventional tissue sections, J.Natl.Cancer Inst. 57: 11-22.

7.Goldenberg D.M.[1978] Immunodiagnosis and immunodetection of colorectal cancer, Cancer Bull. 30: (6) 213-218.

8.Goldenberg D.M. et al.[1978] Use of radiolabelled antibodies to carcinoembryonic antigen for the detection and localization of diverse cancers by external photoscanning, N.Engl.J.Med.298, 1384-1388.

9.Mach J.P. et al.[1980] Tumour Localization or radiolabelled antibodies against carcinoembryonic antigen in patients with carcinoma N.Engl.J.Med. 303, 5-10.

10.Mach J.P. et al.[1978] In vivo localization of anti-CEA antibody in colon carcinoma. Can the results obtained in the nude mice model be extrapolated to the patient situation?. Eur.J. Cancer 1. 113-120.

11.Reif A.E. et al.[1974] Trial of radiolabelled antibody localization in metastases of a patient with tumour containing carcinoembryonic antigen (CEA) J.Surg.Oncol.6,133-150.

12.Primus F.J. et al.[1980] Circulating immune complexes in cancer patients receiving goat radiolocalising antibodies to carcinoembryonic antigen, Cancer Res.40, 497-501.

13.Primus F.J. and Goldenberg D.M.[1980] Immunological considerations in the use of goat antibodies to carcinoembryonic antigen for the radioimmunodetection of cancer, Cancer Res,. 40,2979-2983.

14.Goldenberg D.M. et al.[1980] Radioimmunodetection of cancer with radioactive antibodies to carcinoembryonic antigen, Cancer Res, 40,2984-2992.

15.DeLand F.H. and Goldenberg D.M.[1986] Radiolabelled antibodies: radiochemistry and clinical applications, in L.M. Freeman (ed.) Freeman and Johnson's Clinical Radionuclide Imaging,Grune & Stratton Inc. Orlando pp.1915-1992.

16.Goldenberg D.M. et al[1983] Carcinoembryonic antigen radioimmunodetection in the evaluation of colorectal cancer and in the detection of occult neoplasms, Gastroenterol. 84, 524-532.

17.Larson S.M.[1978-1988] Clinical radioimmunodetection.overview and suggestions for standardisation of clinical trials, Cancer.Res. 50.892-898.

18.Goldenberg D.M.[1988] Targeting of cancer with radiolabelled antibodies: prospects for imaging and therapy, Arch.Path.Lab Med. 112. 580-587.

19.Goldenberg D.M.[1988] Future role of radiolabelled antibodies in oncologic diagnosis and therapy, Semin.Nucl.Med. 19.332-339.

20.Maguire R.T. et al.[1989] Immunoscintigraphy of colorectal adenocarcinoma: results with site-specifically radiolabelled B72.3 (111-In-CYT-103)Antibody Immunocon.Radiopharm. 2.257-269.

21.Delaloye B. et al.[1986] Detection of colorectal carcinoma by emission-computerised tomography after injection of 123-I-labelled Fab or F(ab')2 fragments from monoclonal anti-carcinoembryonicantigen antibodies. J.Clin.Invest.77,301-311.

22.Bischof-delaloyeA et al.[1989] Clinical value of immunoscintigraphyin colorectal carcinoma patients: a prospective trial.J.Nucl.Med.30.1646-1656.

23.Goldenberg D.M. Goldenberg H. et al.[1990] Clinical studies of cancer radioimmunodetectionwith carcinoembryonicantigen monoclonal antibody fragments labelled with 123-I or 99m-Tc, Cancer Res; 50, 909-921.

24.Blumenthal R.D. et al.[1990] Current perspectives and challenges in the use of monoclonal antibodies as imaging and therapeutic agents, Adv.Drug.Del Rev. 4, 279--318.

25.Colcher D. et al.[1990] In vivo tumour targeting of a recombinant single-chain antigen-binding protein,J.Natl.CancerInst., 82, 1191-1198.

26.Siccardi A.G. et al.[1989] Immunoscintigraphyof adenocarcinomasby means of radiolabelled F(ab')2 fragments of an anti-carcinoembryonicantigen monoclonal antibody: a multicentre study, Cancer Res.49, 3095-3103.

27.Baum R.P.et al.[1989] 99m-Tc-labelled anti-CEA monoclonal antibody for tumour immunoscintigraphy:first clinical results, Nucl.Med.Comm. 10, 345-352.

28.Patt Y.Z. et al.[1990] Imaging with indium 111-labelled anticarcinoembryonic antigen monoclonal antibody ZCE-025 of recurrent colorectal or carcinoembryonic antigen-producing cancer in patients with rising serum carcinoembryonic antigen levels and occult metastases.J.Clin.Oncol.8,1246-1254.

29.Abdel-Nabi. et al.[1990] In-111-labelled monoclonal antibody immunoscintigraphy in colorectal carcinoma:safety,sensitivity and preliminary clinical results. Radiology. 175, 163-171.

30.Fairweather D.S. et al.[1983] Improved tumour localisation using indium 111-labelled antibodies, Br.Med.J. 287, 167-170.

31.Patt Y.Z. et al.[1988] Improved tumour localisation with increasing dose of indium-111-labelled anti-carcinoembryonicantigen monoclonalantibodyZCE-025 in metastaticcolorectal cancer. J.Clin.Oncol.6, 1220-1230.

32.Pettit W.A. et al.[1980] Improved protein labelling by stannous tartrate reduction of pertechnetate,J.Nucl.Med.21,59-62.

33.Steenbeck L. and Markwardt J.[1985] Moglichkeiten des einsatzes von monoklonalen Antikorpern gegen CEA in der szintigrafishe tumordiagnostik, Arch.Geschwulstforsch,55, 207-214.

34.Schwarz A. and Steinstrasser A.[1987] A novel approach to Tc-99m labelled monoclonal antibodies. J.Nucl.Med.28, 721.

35.Hansen H.J. et al.[1990] Preclinical evaluation of an "instant" 99m-Tc labelling kit for antibody imaging. Cancer Res.50, 794-798.

36.Goldenberg D.M. et al. [1990] Imaging of colorectal carcinoma with radiolabelled antibodies.Semin.Nucl.Med.19,262-281.

37.Hansen H.J. et al.[1990] Site-specific direct labelling of monoclonal antibodies with technetium and rhenium isotopes for the improved imaging and therapy of cancer, submitted for publication.

38.Larson S.M. et al. [1983] Localisation of 131-I-labelled p97-specific Fab fragments in human melanoma as a basis for radiotherapy.J.Clin.Invest,72,2102-2114.

39.Order S.E. et al.[1989] Current status of radioimmunoglobulinsin the treatment of human malignancy,Oncology3, 115-120.

40.Dykes P.W. et al. [1987] Radioimmunotherapyof cancer: clinical studies and limiting factors, Cancer Treat.Rev.14,87-106.

41.Epenetos A.A. et al.[1986] Limitationsof radiolabelledmonoclonalantibodiesfor localisation of human neoplasms,Cancer Res. 46,3183-3191.

42.Order S.E. et al.[1985] Iodine-131 antiferritin, a new treatment modality in hepatoma: a Radiation Therapy Oncology Group study, J.Clin.Oncol.3, 1573-1582.

43.Lenhard R.E. et al.[1985]Isotopic immunoglobulin: a new system therapy for advanced Hodgkin's disease, J.Clin.Oncol. 3, 1296-1300.

44.Rosen S.T. et al.[1989] Progress in the treatment of cutaneous T cell lymphomas with radiolabelled monoclonal antibodies, Nucl.Med.Biol. 16, 667-668.

45.DeNardo S.J. et al.[1988] Treatment of B cell malignancies with 131-I Lym-1 monoclonal antibodies, Int.J.Cancer,Suppl.3,96-101.

46.Press O.W. et al.[1989] Treatment of refractorynon-Hodgkin's lymphoma with radiolabelled MB-1 (anti-CD37) antibody.J.Clin.Oncol.7,1027-1038.

47.Goldenberg D.M. et al.[1990] Targeting dosimetry and radioimmunotherapy of B-cell lymphomas with 131-I-labelled LL2 (EPB-2) monoclonal antibody, submitted for publication.

48.Schroff R. et al.[1985] Human anti-murine immunoglobulin responses in patients receiving monoclonal antibody therapy, Cancer Res. 45,879-885.

49.Pawlak-Byczkowskaet al.[1989] Two new monoclonal antibodies, EPB-1 and EPB-2, reactive with human lymphoma,Cancer Res.49, 4568-4577.

50.Sharkey R.M. et al.[1988] Radioimmunotherapyof human xenografts with 90-Y-labelled monoclonal antibodies to carcinoembryonicantigen, Cancer Res.48, 3270-3275.

51.Moi M.K. et al.[1990] Stable bifunctional chelates of metals used in radiotherapy, Cancer Res.50, 789-793.

52.Gansow O.S. et al.[1990] Chelates and antibodies: current methods and new directions in D.M. Goldenberg (ed) Cancer imaging with Radiolabelled Antibodies, Kluwer Publ.Norwell, MA.pp153-172.

53.Cole W.C. et al.[1986] Serum stability of Cu-67 chelates: comparison with 111-In and 57-Co Nucl.Med.Biol.13, 363-368.

54.Deutsch E. et al.[1986] The chemistry of rhenium and technetium as related to the use of isotopes of these elements in therapeutic and diagnostic nuclear medicine,Nucl.Med.Biol. 13,465-477.

55.Kozak R.W. et al.[1986] Bismuth-212-labelledanti-Tac monoclonal antibody: alpha-particle-emittingradionuclidesas modalitiesfor radioimmunotherapy,Proc.Natl.Acad.Sci.USA 83,474-478.

56.Vaughan A.T.M. et al.[1982] The in vivo fate of a 111-At labelled monoclonal antibody with known specificity in a murine system. Int.J.Rad.Oncol.Biol.Phy.8,1943-1946.

57.James K.[1990] Human monoclonal antibodies and engineer antibodies in the management of cancer,Semin.CancerBiol.1,243-253.

58.Shar D.R. et al.[1988] Mouse/human chimeric antibodies to a tumour associated antigen: biologic activity of the four human IgG subclasses, J.Natl.Cancer Inst.80, 1553-1559.

59.Blumenthal R.D. et al.[1988] Reduction of radioantibody-induced myelotoxicity by recombinant interleukin-1, Cancer Res. 48, 5403-5406.

60.Blumenthal R.D. et al.[1990] Use of hematopoietic growth factors to control myelosuppressioncaused by radioimmunotherapy,Cancer Res.50, 1003-1007.

EVALUATION OF THE DIAGNOSTIC UTILITY OF IMMUNOSCINTIGRAPHY IN ONCOLOGY

G.L. Buraggi

Abstract

The requirementsfor the routine use of radioimmunoscintigraphy(RIS) of cancer in clinical practice are realised and discussed. Imaging quality, performance, feasibility and clinical utility of these examinations are the most important factors to be considered. The results obtained so far by the study of a large number of patients are very good and it seems important, for the development of these methods to widen the field of clinical applications both with new prospective trials and with extensive use of RIS in daily routine.

Introduction

The aim of this paper is to analyse and discuss, with particular reference to our own experience, the requirementsfor routine use of immunoscintigraphy(RIS) of tumours in clinical practice and to evaluate the diagnostic utility of these methods in comparison with the results obtained with other diagnostic procedures available in clinical oncology for screening, diagnosis, prognosis and monitoring. Radio-immunoscintigraphycan be classified among the imaging methods, even if image generation in this case is based not only on the physical properties of the radiation used but especially on the biological phenomena involving a specific immunological reaction.

The requirements for the use of imaging methods in clinical practice can be summarised

R. P. Baum et al. (eds.), Clinical Use of Antibodies, 15–30.

as follows:- high imaging quality, simplicity of execution, no risk for the patient, acceptable cost, high diagnostic efficacy. In particular if we want to evaluate an immunoscintigraphic technique it seems appropriate to consider:

- the quality of the tumour image obtained
- the performance of the technique
- the feasibility of the examination in clinical practice
- the clinical utility deriving from its application

The Tumour Image

Several factors, which determine tumour uptake and biodistribution of the immunoreagent, contribute to generate the tumour image.

A more extensive analysis of these factors was reported in previous papers (1, 2); I will only report here some of the practical conclusions about tumour uptake, biodistribution of the radioimmunoreagent and image generation.

First of all, it should be remembered that the intensity of the image representation is directly related to the intensity of the signal which in turn, is directly related to the value of the total radioactivity present in the tumour and this corresponds to the radioactive concentration multiplied by the volume. Therefore, the volume of a tumour and the concentration of the radioactivity are only indirectly related to the scintigraphic result. This means that with sufficient radioactivity it is possible to detect even a punctual source. Conversely, when the total activity is too low, even large tumours are not imaged.

This behaviour can explain the results obtained in the detection of melanoma lesions of different sizes as reported in Table 1.

TABLE 1. Correlation between scintigraphic results and size of melanoma lesions

SIZE (CM)	POSITIVE N°	NEGATIVE N°	TOTAL N°
≤1	4	8	12
2	16	5	21
3	14	0	14
4	7	3	10
≥5	13	4	17
TOTAL	54 (73%)	20 (27%)	74

As can be seen, the best results were obtained in the detection of lesions >1cm. Nevertheless, although it is true that small lesions are more frequently missed, several tumours of large volume were not detected either.

As to the image contrast, there is a good correlation of this parameter and the ratio between the radioactivity of tumour and background (T/B). In our experience, the maximum T/B ratio in human subjects does not exceed 6 or 7. By contrast, when using the same immunoreagents in animal models, we found T/B ratio values as high as 40-50 (3).

It is also worth noticing that the values of this index and its variations with time are often different for the same antigen-antibody system, not only in different patients but also in different neoplastic localisations in the same patient (4).

This phenomenon is due not only to the different activity present in different cases in tumour and background but also to the different trend of its variations.

From a practical point of view, it is important to establish a correlation between the values of T/B ratio and the results available. In Table 2 the scintigraphic results obtained in a series of patients bearing colo-rectal tumours of about the same size are compared with the T/B ratio values.

TABLE 2. Radioimmunodetection of colo-rectal carcinoma with F023C5 MAb comparison between tumor/background ratio (T/B) and results

PATIENT	T/B	IMMUNOSCINTIGRAPHY
1	4.9	+
2	2.9	+
3	2.6	+
4	2.6	+
5	2.0	+
6	1.9	+
7	1.9	+
8	1.8	+
9	1.6	+
10	1.5	+
11	1.5	+
12	1.4	+
13	1.3	±
14	1.3	±
15	1.0	-
16	1.0	-
17	1.0	-

Radioimmunodetectionwas performed with an anti-CEA antibody. For values higher than 1.4, suitable tumour imaging was obtained. Doubtful results were obtained for the value 1.3. For a T/B ratio inferior to 1.3 negative results were obtained (5). A positive immunoscintigraphic result depends also on the site where the tumour is located. Several anatomic and biological factors contribute to determine this result. For example, Fig.1 reports the sensitivity obtained in the detection of melanoma localisations in different organs. The sensitivity decreases from localisations in the nymph nodes, brain, skin to those in the lungs and liver (6, 7).

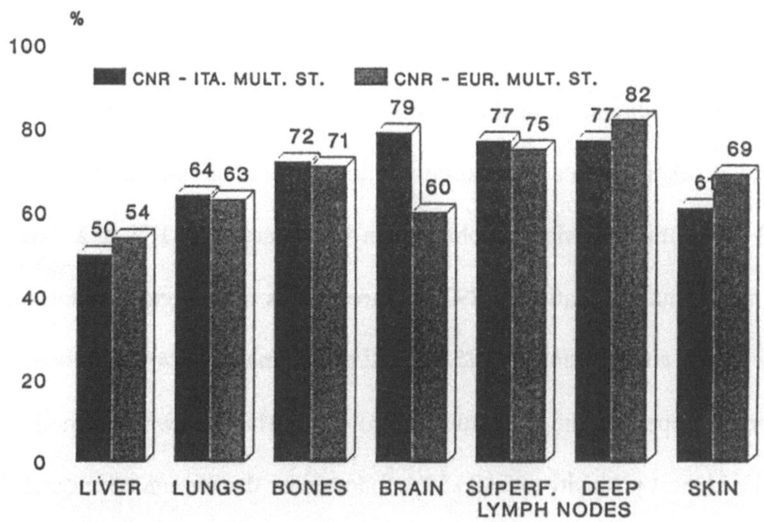

Fig.1 Radioimmunodetection of melanoma sensitivity for different lesion site (539 in 254 patients)

The imaging quality can be improved in different ways. For instance, by using a pure gamma emitter like 123-I or 99mTc, it is possible to administer higher amounts of radioactivity without increasing the radiation burden to the patient (8, 9, 10). Thus, a high signal is obtained, with an energy more suitable to the instruments in use.

The use of SPECT also allows an important improvement of tumour uptake (11-12). There are different methods to reduce the interference of background, for example, dual isotope subtraction, biological background reduction or, more interesting, the probability mapping method proposed and used by Granowska et al (13).

Other methods, now under study such as the avidin-biotin technique, will probably also be useful to improve imaging quality (14).

The Performance

The performance of an immunoscintigraphic technique is essential to evaluate its diagnostic importance. I will discuss here the results obtained in several studies performed at our Institute and at other Centres as cooperative multicentre trials (4-9, 15-20).

Table 3 shows the positivity rate obtained in the detection by RIS of a large number of malignant melanoma localisations (1290) in three series of patients: a pilot study and two multicentre clinical studies using the 225.28S anti melanoma monoclonal antibody labelled with different radioisotopes. In the pilot study the compound labelled with technetium allowed us to obtain the highest positivity rate (86.7%), followed by the indium compound (76.6%) and by the three immunoreagents labelled with 131-I and 123-I (56.5%). The mean sensitivity was 73%.

TRIAL	PATIENTS	LESIONS	POSITIVITY RATE (%)			
			^{131}I-^{123}I	^{111}IN	^{99m}Tc	OVERALL
PILOTE	42	74	56.5	76.6	8 .7	73
ITALIAN MULTICENTER	254	539	-	59	74	70
EUROPEAN MULTICENTER	493	728	-	-	70	70

Table 3. Immunoscintigraphy of malignant melanoma: pilot and CNR multicentre trials positivity rate obtained in detection of 1290 tumour localisations

No false-positive results were observed.

The positivity rate obtained in a multicentre study, including 10 Italian nuclear medicine centres (6), shows the same trend when comparing the compounds labelled with indium and technetium. Positivity rates of 59% for indium and of 74% for technetium were found. The mean positivity rate was 70%. It is interesting to point out that, in this series, 82% of the lesions >2cm were imaged, but also 59% of the lesions of 2cm or less. Finally, the positivity rate obtained in a multicentre study performed with the cooperation of 20 European centres using technetium labelled reagent was 70%. Whereas the mean sensitivity was about the same in the three series, a difference was seen between the positivity rates obtained with the immunoreagent labelled with 99mTc.

This is probably due to different factors, and especially to the different composition of the series examined (site and size of the lesions) and the different instruments used by the single groups. The cumulative results obtained in the three series included in a study of 751 melanoma patients are reported in Table 4.

TABLE 4. Immunoscintigraphy of malignant melanoma: CNR multicenter trials overall results in 751 patients*

	N°	%
SENSITIVITY	461/569	81
SPECIFICITY	173/182	95
ACCURACY	634/751	84
PREDICTIVE VALUE		
OF POSITIVE RESULT	461/470	98
OF NEGATIVE RESULT	173/281	61

*POSITIVE RESULT: AT LEAST 1 LESION IMAGED

Patients with at least 1 lesion imaged were classified as positive. Good sensitivity and accuracy were obtained, but the high specificity and the high predictive value of the positive results obtained are of most interest for the clinical application of RIS, especially considering the fact that several other examinations routinely used in clinical oncology show lower values of these indexes.

Good results were obtained also with the use of the FO23C5 anti-CEA antibody in the study of gastrointestinal and non-gastrointestinaltumours.

Table 5 reports the positivity rate obtained in gastrointestinal cancer in a pilot and a multicentre study including 11 Italian centres (10).

The best results were seen in a study of primary tumours and especially of local relapses, with a positivity rate of 90%.

TABLE 5. Immunoscintigraphy of colo-rectal carcinoma with FO23C5 anti-CEA antibody positivity rate obtained in pilot and CNR multicenter trials

TRIAL	PATIENTS	LESIONS	POSITIVITY RATE (%)				
			PRIMARY	LOCAL RELAPSES	P+LR	LIVER	OVERAL
PILOTE	51	64	64	90	-	25	64
MULTICENTER	254	486	-	-	75	52	76

Results were poorest, in the detection of liver metastases.

Table 6 reports the cumulative results of these studies, which allow us to confirm that, also with this antibody, the most relevant finding consists in the high specificity and the high predictive value of the positive test for both series of tumours.

TABLE 6. Immunoscintigraphy with F023C5 anti-CEA antibody overall results in 480 patients

TUMORS	GASTROINTESTINAL (277 PTS) %	NON-GASTROINTESTINAL (203 PTS) %	TOTAL (480 PTS) %
SENSITIVITY	78	81	79
SPECIFICITY	95	97	96
ACCURACY	80	83	81
PREDICTIVE VALUE			
POSITIVE RESULT	99	99	99

The predictive value of the negative results was doubtful due to the small number of truly negative patients examined in comparison with the relatively high number of false-negative results observed.

Our results with immunoscintigraphyof ovarian carcinoma using both OC 125 and MOv18 - are also good, even if a smaller number of patients was examined. With the MOv18 antibody, higher values of the positivity rate were obtained in the detection of pelvic lesions (80%) in comparison to those localised in the abdomen (61%) and this behaviour was observed also with the OC 125 antibody.

Only the results obtained or directly verified by ourselves are reported here, but similar favourable results were reported by many other authors (23-28) and I think that we may conclude that the performance of the majority of these examinations is very good.

The Feasibility

As to the feasibility of immunoscintigraphic techniques, it is possible to say that the execution of the test does not cause any special inconvenience to the patient. The test requires those instruments and scintigraphic techniques that are currently in use. Examinations can be completed during the first day if 99mTc or 123-I are used and require 2-4 days if other nuclides are used.

As to adverse reactions it should be underlined that only one patient among about 1500 studied in the trials reported here, complained of a reaction consisting of a cutting pain in the lower back and epigastric region that subsided in one hour without any therapy. About the same frequency (0.09%) is reported in the literature (29,30).

Dosimetric evaluations show that the radiation burden to the patient is comparable to that of other nuclear medicine examinations. Some radio-immunoreagents required for immunoscintigraphy are readily available as commercial radiopharmaceuticals. Nevertheless, a larger industrial production is to be hoped for.

Another problem is represented by the generation of human antimurine antibodies (HAMA) by the patient, after injection of an immunoreagent of murine origin. No correlation has been demonstrated between high serum levels of HAMA and adverse reactions. Nevertheless, circulating HAMA may react with radiolabelled antibodies and reduce the possibility to obtain suitable tumour imaging.

Table 7 shows the result obtained by Seccamani et al.in patients injected once or several times with monoclonal antibodies of murine origin for radioimmunoscintigraphy or radioimmunotherapy(31). It can be seen that the incidence of high HAMA levels in serum is very low after injection of F(ab')2 fragments even if repeated several times.The incidence increases when the whole IgG is used,especially for therapeutical purposes which require higher amounts of immunoglobulins.

TABLE 7. HAMA levels in patients sera (from Seccamani et al.)(31)

GROUP	IMMUNOREAGENT INJECTED	SINGLE DOSE	PT. N°	NEG. N°	POS. N°
A	FAB' ONCE	350 UG	15	15	0
B	F(AB')2 ONCE	250-500 UG	123	120	3
C	F(AB')2 TWICE	"	31	26	5
D	F(AB')2 3 TIMES	"	14	10	4
E	F(AB')2 4 TIMES	"	6	4	2
F	IGG ONCE	1 MG	40	32	8
G	IGG TWICE	"	5	2	3
H	IGG 3 TIMES	"	5	0	5
I	IGG ONCE FOR THERAPY	20-50 MG	10	2	8
L	IGG TWICE FOR THERAPY	"	6	1	5
M	IGG 3 TIMES FOR THERAPY	"	4	0	4
N	IGG 4 TIMES FOR THERAPY	"	3	0	3
O	IGG 5 TIMES FOR THERAPY	"	1	0	1
P	IGG 6 TIMES FOR THERAPY	"	2	0	2

The Clinical Utility

The clinical utility of an examination should be evaluated in terms of its diagnostic efficacy compared to the results obtained with other diagnostic methods used.

At present, immunoscintigraphy can be very useful in the following situations:

- detection of regional or metastatic invasion of primary tumour
- early detection of tumour relapses during follow-up
- differentiation between benign and malignant lesions
- detection of new unexpected lesions in advanced disease

I shall give some examples of these applications.

In clinical practice there are often difficulties in the diagnosis of lymphatic involvement in patients with primary melanoma and regional lymphnode enlargement. A comparative clinical and scintigraphic prospective study was performed in 44 patients (32).

As can be seen in Table 8, although the sensitivity of the clinical examination is high, immunoscintigraphy shows higher values of all the other indexes and particularly of the sensitivity and predictive value of the positive result.

The high sensitivity observed in the detection of local relapses of colorectal cancer induced us to perform a prospective trial in a series of 59 patients, in order to compare the results obtained with immunoscintigraphy with those obtained in the same patients with CT scan, magnetic resonance (MRI) and ultrasound (US) (table 9) (33).

TABLE 8. Immunoscintigraphy of melanoma: prospective study comparative results obtained with clinical evaluation and immunoscintigraphy in 44 patients with suspect lymphnode involvement

	CLINICAL EVALUATION	IMMUNOSCINTIGRAPHY
SENSITIVITY	86	76
SPECIFICITY	67	100
ACCURACY	82	87
PREDICTIVE VALUE		
OF POSITIVE RESULT	89	100
OF NEGATIVE RESULT	60	78

TABLE 9. Immunoscintigraphy with anti-CEA F023C5 antibody prospective study on 59 patients with suspect local relapses of colo-rectal cancer: comparison with other diagnostic methods

	RIS	MRI	CT	US
SENSITIVITY	89	93	69	41
SPECIFICITY	79	67	67	78
ACCURACY	86	86	68	54
PREDICTIVE VALUE				
OF POSITIVE RESULTS	93	88	86	78
OF NEGATIVE RESULTS	69	80	42	41

Only MRI showed results as good as those obtained with immunoscintigraphy, whereas the values of the different indexes obtained with CT scan and ultrasound in particular were clearly inferior.

Table 10 reports the incidence of unexpected lesions detected in the three multicentre trials already mentioned in the study of 1245 patients with advanced disease (6,7,15)

TABLE 10. Unexpected lesions detected with immunoscintigraphy in 1245 patients with advanced disease

MULTICENTER STUDY	PATIENTS	LESIONS KNOWN	LESIONS UNEXPECTED	UNEXPECTED LESIONS IN "LESION FREE" PATIENTS
CEA	498	708	218	79 IN 35
MELANOMA ITALIAN	254	412	127	32 IN 15
MELANOMA EUROPEAN	493	605	123	62 IN 42

The number of unexpected lesions was 468 which, in comparison to the 1725 known localisations, is very high. It is interesting to note that 173 lesions were found in the examination of 92 apparently "lesion-free" patients.

In conclusion, the results discussed here are an example, taken from our own experience, of the diagnostic utility of cancer immunoscintigraphyin clinical practice an example that can be confirmed by the results of a large number of trials performed so far.

Certainly, these techniques will be improved by further biological and technical advances, but I think that it is also very important for the development of these methods to widen the field of clinical applications both with new prospective trials and with extensive use of RIS in daily routine.

References

1. Buraggi G.L.[1985] Radioimmunodetectionof Cancer.J.Nucl.Med.All.Sci.29:261-267

2. Buraggi G.L.[1990] Requirementsfor the use of radioimmunodetectionof cancer in clinical practice. In. Goldenberg D.M. [Editor] Cancer Imaging with radiolabelled antibodies. M.Nijhoff Publ.Norwell USA [in press]

3. Ripamonti M. et al [1988] Monoclonal anti-CEA antibody: factors affecting localisation in a preclinical study. In.J.Biol. Markers 3, 249-258

4. Buraggi G.L. et al[2985] Immunoscintigraphywith anti-melanoma monoclonal antibodies. In: Donato L, Britton K.E. [Eds] Immunoscintigraphy. Gordon & Breach Sci.Publ.New York, London pp.215-254

5. Buraggi G.L. et al [1987] Immunoscintigraphyof colorectal carcinoma with F[ab']: fragments of anti-CEA monoclonal antibody. Cancer Det.Prev. 10: 335-345

6. Siccardi A.G. et al [[1986] Multi-centre study of immunoscintigraphy with radiolabelled monoclonal antibodies in patients with melanoma. Cancer Res: 4817-4822

7. Siccardi A.G. et al European Multicentre Study Group [1989] European multicentre study on melanoma immunoscintigraphy by means of 99mTc-labelled monoclonal antibody fragments. Eur.J.Nucl.Med.[in press]

8. Buraggi G.L. et al [1985] Imaging with 131-I labelled monoclonal antibodies to a high-molecular-weightmelanoma-associatedantigen in patients with melanoma: efficacy of whole immunoglobulin and its F[ab']2 fragments. Cancer Res 45: 3378-3387

9. Buraggi G.L. et al [1984] Immunoscintigraphy with 123-I, 99mTc and 111-In labelled F[ab']2 fragments of monoclonal antibodies to a human high molecular weight melanoma-associated antigen. J.Nucl.Med.All Sci. 28: 283-295

10. Baum B. et al [1989] 99mTc labelled anti-CEA monoclonal antibody for tumour immunoscintigraphy: first clinical results Nucl.J.Med.Commun. 10: 345-352

11. Delaloye B. et al [1986] Detection of colorectal carcinoma by emission computerised tomography after injection of 123-I labelled Fab or F[ab']2 fragments from monoclonal anti-carcinoembryonic antigen antibodies. J.Clin Invest. 77: 301-311

12. Bares R. et al [1988] Validity of tomographical methods for radioimmunodetection of gastrointestinal tumours. In: Greten H. Klapdor R. eds. New tumour markers and their monoclonal antibodies - actual clinical relevance for diagnosis and therapy of solid tumours. Thieme, 470-4

13. Granowska M. et al [1988] Kinetic analysis and probability mapping applied to the detection of ovarian cancer by radioimmunoscintigraphy.J.Nucl.Med.29: 599-607

14. Paganelli G. et al [1988] In vivo labelling of biotinylated monoclonal antibodies by radioactive avidin: a strategy to increase tumour radiolocalisation. Int.J.Cancer Suppl. 2: 121-125

15. Siccardi A.G. et al [1989] Immunoscintigraphy of adenocarcinomas by means of radiolabelled F[ab']2 fragments of anti-carcinoembryogenic antigen monoclonal antibody. Cancer Res 49: 3095-3103

16. Buraggi G.L. [1988] Tumour radioimmunodetection by anti-melanoma and anti -CEA monoclonal antibodies: pilot and prospective studies. In: Srivastava S [ed. Radiolabelled monoclonal antibodies for imaging and therapy. Plenum Publ.Corp.New York, London pp.653-681

17. Natali P.G. et al [1984] Serological and binding characteristics of a monoclonal antibody [MoAb] to a human high molecular weight-melanoma associated antigen [HMW-MAA] for tumour imaging. In: Giraldo G. et al [eds] from Oncogenes to Tumour Antigens. Elsevier, Amsterdam pp.127-134

18. Buraggi G.L. et al [1986] Radioimmunodetection of malignant melanoma with radiolabelled 131-I, 123-I, 111-In, 99mTc monoclonal antibodies and F[ab']2 fragments. In: Winkler C [ed] Nuclear Medicine in Clinical Oncology. Springer Verlag. Berlin, Heidelberg, New York, pp.207-214

19. Buraggi G.L. Gasparini M [1989] Immunoscintigraphy of melanoma using radiolabelled antibodies: pilot, prospective studies and Italian multicentre clinical trials. Nucl.Med.Biol.16: 629-632

20. Buraggi G.L. Gasparini M [1989] Immunoscintigraphy of malignant melanoma In Chatal Y.F. [ed] Monoclonal antibodies in immunoscintigraphy. CRC Press USA p.259-273

21. Buraggi G.L. et al [1988] In: A new monoclonal antibody [MOv18] against ovarian cancer for imaging and therapy. Hoofer R. Bergaun H [eds] Radioactive Isotopes in Clinical Medicine and Research. Schattauer. Stuttgart p.57-62

22. Crippa F. et al [1990] Clinical value of radioimmunoscintigraphy in the follow-up of ovarian carcinoma: a prospective study. Accepted by Int.J.Biol Markers.

23. Chatal J.F. et al [1987] Immunoscintigraphy of recurrences of gynecological carcinomas. J.Nucl.Med.28: 1807-1819

24. Bischof-Delaloye A. et al [1989] Clinical value of immunoscintigraphy in colorectal carcinoma patients: a prospective study. J.Nucl.Med.30, 1646-1656

25. Granowska M. et al [1984] Ovarian cancer: diagnosis using 123-I monoclonal antibody in comparison with surgical findings. Nucl.Med.Commun.5: 485-99

26. Baum R.P. et al [1987] Clinical results of immunoscintigraphy and radioimmunotherapy. Nucl Med.26.68-78.

27. Goldenberg D.M. [1989] Future role of radiolabelled monoclonal antibodies in oncological diagnosis and therapy. Sem.Nucl.Med.19:332-339

28. Goldenberg D.M. et al [1989] Imaging of colorectal carcinoma with radiolabelled antibodies Sem.Nucl.Med.19:262-281

29. Britton K.E. et al [1989] A brief guide to the practice of radioimmunoscintigraphyand radioimmunotherapyin cancer. Int.J.Biol.Markers 4: 106-118

30. Cascinelli N. et al [1988] Anti-melanoma monoclonal antibody 225-28S: evaluation of toxicity in man. Tumori 4: 35-40

31. Seccamani E et al [1989] Specificity of human immunoglobulin response to murine monoclonal antibodies. In:Schmidt HAE, Buraggi G.L. [eds] Nuclear Medicine: trends and possibilities in Nuclear Medicine Schattauer. Stuttgart p. 67-670

32. Buraggi G.L. et al [1986] Radioimmunodetectionof melanoma: preliminary results of a prospective study. In.J.Biol.Markers 1: 47-54

33. Gasparini M [1988] Tumour imaging of colo-rectal carcinoma with an anti-CEA monoclonal antibody. Int.J.Cancer: Suppl 2: 81-84

THE QUALITY CONTROL AND CLINICAL TESTING OF RADIOLABELLED ANTIBODIES

Peter.H. Cox and Knud Kristensen

Introduction

Within the European context any preparation which is compounded,in a hospital, for administrationto Humans for medicinal purposes,isthe responsibilityof the Hospital Pharmacist with respect to its efficacy and safety in use (1). Radiopharmaceuticals fall within this definition. Similarly the prescribing Physician is responsible for administering the preparation to the patient and as such is also responsible for the quality of care which is given.

To meet these responsibilitiesit is obviously necessaryto develop quality control procedures which will define the physico-chemical nature of the product and its stability to ensure a reproduciblebiodistribution. Prior to clinical use toxicological and biodistributionstudies must be carried out in animals followed by a limited phase one study in humans to determine that biodistribution patterns are essentially the same as in animals. All of this may indeed be difficult to realise in the case of monoclonal antibodies because of the lack of suitable animal models.

With respect to this clinical trials become a very important part of the development phase of a new labelled antibody but may be difficult to implement because of the ethical considerations. Good planning is therefore essential to ensure that optimal information is obtained to define the characteristicsof the labelled antibody to provide data for registration purposes or in the case of Hospital based products to provide supporting evidence of safety and efficacy in use.The aquisition of this informationshould be seen as a continuous process which should be followed up well into the period when the product has been accepted for routine use.

Labelled antibodies are particularly complicated because we are concerned with three differentsets of criteria namely: As a radioactivesubstance,as a Pharmaceuticaland as a Blood Product (Vaccines and Sera).

R. P. Baum et al. (eds.), Clinical Use of Antibodies, 31–35.

Product Definition

The characteristics of a Radiopharmaceutical are determined by the use of a standardised preparation method using raw materials of clearly specified quality. The physical chemical characteristics of the final product are determined by the quality control procedures and specifications which are laid down. The combination of these factors will determine the reproducibility of the biodistribution of the radiopharmaceutical.

In the case of monoclonal antibodies the method of raising the antibody and the origin of the original source are important and should be recorded. Experience has shown that such information may be lost especially in the case of antibodies from non commercial sources (2). The production of antibodies should be carried out in accordance with official guidelines for Good Manufacturing Practice (3).

A potential source of problems with respect to this is the fact that many of the antibodies in current use are raised using the murine ascites model and not from cell culture. There are ethical objections to this from the point of view of Animal Rights and a number of countries have either taken official or voluntary action to eliminate this method of production (4).

Specifications

Let us now consider the specifications required for a radiopharmaceutical based upon an antibody as carrier molecule. These will apply to both ready labelled antibody i.e. supplied ready for injection and to in house labelling.

1) **Labelling Kit and Final Product:**

Identity:

Antibody (source and production method)

Conjugating Agent

Radionuclide

Adjuvents (Buffer, Support Material for freeze drying etc)

Potency:

Immunoreactivity

Radionuclide Concentration Specific activity

Protein concentration

Purity:

Radiochemical purity

Aggregation

Extraneous proteins i.e.DNA

Chemical impurities (arising from conjugating material,reagents used to produce fragmentation,labellingaids etc.)

Sterility

Pyrogens

Murine viruses

Stability:

In Vitro

In Vivo

2) Radioactive solution for labelling

Identity:

Radionuclide characteristics

Potency:

Radionuclide concentration

Purity:

Radionuclide purity

Radiochemical purity

Specific activity

Chemical composition

Chemical impurities [heavy metal ions,reducing substances]

Stability:

In Vitro

Suitable analytical methods for each parameter must be developed together with limiting values which the product must satisfy. Such limits may have to be defined after practical experience from a number of batch preparations has been obtained. This may be difficult with reference to the antibody itself since it may only have been raised upon one occasion. When the final product form has been fully developed different parameters of the production and a number of the analytical procedures may still require validation.

Safety Testing

The safety testing of a radioactive immunoreactive product poses special problems. Because of the low chemical concentrations involved it is practically impossible to carry out objective acute toxicity studies. The possibility of making accurate predictions of the possible incidence and nature of immunologically based adverse reactions in humans is also difficult without human data.

Nevertheless it is necessary to carry out some form of safety evaluation proir to administration of the product to humans. Basic elements of this are single dose toxicity in two animal species [one non rodent] in in vitro cross reactivity. Guidance can be obtained from Draft EEC Guidelines and other relevant publications (5-8). All studies should be carried out in accordance with Good Laboratory Practice Guidelines (9). Radiation dosimetry estimates are a particular problem (10) with antibodies because the relevant pharmacokinetic data required may not be available until the first human studies have been made. It is therefore essential to record detailed observations concerning the biodistribution, excretion and eventual side effects, including possible HAMA development, from the first patient series.

Efficacy

Animal models relevant to human disease states may not be available. It is, however, good practice to test a new complex in as relevant a biological model as possible before human use. Furthermore in vitro data from immunocytochemistry and binding studies with labelled material should also be taken into account.

When considering the aquisition of biodistribution data in humans it should be remembered that the EEC guidelines do not recommend the administration of labelled antibodies to normal subjects but that data should be obtained from genuine patients.

Conclusions

At the present time there are no official regulations as to precisely what data is required prior to commencing clinical trials with labelled antibodies in humans. In general the regulations concerning radiopharmaceuticals apply and the concept guidelines (2,7) concerning antibodies in particular are being used already by several national authorities. The Concept EEC guidelines stress that they are not designed to deal with clinical trial material but nevertheless studies should be designed, and data collected, in a systematic manner to provide the information necessary to establish efficacy and safety in use (11).

References

1. Product liability and the Pharmacist (1986) Pharm.J.237.744-745.

2. On the production and quality control of monoclonal antibodies of murine origin intended for use in man. EEC III 1859/86-EW, June 1987 Rev 7, Final.

3. Guide to Good ManufacturingPractice for Medicinal Products. EEC III/2244/87-EN,June 1988,Rev 5.

4. Monoclonal Antibodies: In vivo and In vitro production on a laboratory scale,with considerationof the legal aspects of Animal protection.KuhlmannI. Kurth W. and Ruhdel I. (1989) ATLA 17.73-82.

5. On the preclinicalbiologicalsafetytestingof medicinal productsderived from biotechnology. EEC III/407/87-EN June 1988, Rev 5.

6. The joint task group on clinical utility of labelled antibodies of the Nuclear Medical Society Europe [SNME] and the European Nuclear Medicine Society. (1986) Int.J.Biol.Markers.1.147-153.

7. Working party on clinical use of antibodies. Operation manual for control of production,preclinical toxicology and Phase I trial of anti tumour antibodies and drug antibody conjugates.(1986)Brit.J.Cancer.54.557-568.

8. Points to consider in the manufacture and testing of monoclonal antibody products for human use.(1987) Dept of Health and Human Services USA June 1.

9. Good Laboratory Practice. OECD,C(81) 30 Final, May 12.1981.

10. Radiation dose to patients from Radiopharmaceuticals,(1987) ICRP 53. Annals of the ICRP.18.1-4.

11. Radiopharmaceuticals.DrugApplication Nordic Guidelines. (1988) NLN Publ.

CLINICAL UTILITY OF RADIOLABELLED MONOCLONAL ANTIBODIES IN THE MANAGEMENT OF GASTROINTESTINAL CANCER

J.F. Chatal, A. Chetanneau, P. Peltier, C. Curtet and P.A. Lehur.

INTRODUCTION

More than 10 years have gone by since the first use of radiolabelled monoclonal antibodies in oncological scintigraphic imaging (1). This period might seem adequate to allow a new technique to acquire full maturity and take its place in routine use among the other conventionalimaging methods, (ultrasonography,computed tomographyand magneticresonance imaging). However, immunoscintigraphy has not reached this stage of routine clinical use, particularly in the diagnostic evaluation of colorectal cancers. It would thus seem useful to analyze the reasons for this delay and to consider the real clinical utility of this new approach and its future prospects at short and middle term.

Diagnosis by scintigraphic imaging can be complimented by intraoperative detection using a hand held probe, a procedure referred to as radioimmunoguidedsurgery, which is performed a few days after injection of an antibody. This original approach has also been under evaluation for several years, particularly in the United States (2), and it is time to assess results and determine what its role will be as whether its clinical utility has been clearly demonstrated.

The purpose of this report was thus to define the utility today of radiolabelled monoclonal antibodies in the diagnostic evaluation of colorectal carcinomas and to envisage the probable technological development at short and middle term.

Is a New In Vivo Diagnostic Method Necessary to Evaluate the Course of Colorectal Carcinoma?

Diagnosis of primary colorectal carcinoma is exclusively endoscopic, and imaging techniques play no role in this indication. Once the histopathologic diagnosis has been demonstrated, preoperative ultrasonography can be useful to determine the spread of the carcinoma, particularly in the liver. In fact, the real diagnosis of the spread of the disease is reached during surgery to achieve macroscopically complete tumour resection when possible or, in case of an extensive cancer, palliative treatment to improve patient comfort. Up to this stage in the

R. P. Baum et al. (eds.), Clinical Use of Antibodies, 37–44.

disease, imaging techniques - and particularly immunoscintigraphy- thus have no determinant clinical utility.

When tumour resection has apparently been complete, it is necessary to monitor the patient regularly by serial serum assays of tumour markers, including the carcinoembryonic antigen (CEA) and CA 19-9 antigen, so that a possible recurrence can be detected as early as possible. In the event of an elevation in one of these markers (mainly CEA), confirmed by a second assay within a short time, there must be proof of suspected recurrence before second-look surgery can be considered. It has been clearly demonstrated that tumour-marker-guided early resection of a recurrence is beneficial to the patient in terms of comfort and survival. The aim of efficient monitoring after resection of a primary colorectal cancer is thus to detect a recurrence early by means of tumour marker assays. In the case of marker elevation, the chances of performing complete resectability must be determined in order to avoid another operation that would be useless for a patient whose tumour involvement is too great. Only 50% of patients had completely resectable recurrences (mainly isolated local ones) when the decision to perform second-look surgery was based solely on an elevation in CEA serum concentration (3). The CT scan can help identify patients with a resectable tumour who could benefit from second-look surgery. Unfortunately, this imaging technique underestimates the volume of disease, falsely indicating a need for surgery in patients whose recurrence is already too large to be efficiently resected (4). The CT scan can thus be usefully complemented by immunoscintigraphy which, after several years of methodological advances, has given proof of generally greater efficiency than other imaging techniques.

Immunoscintigraphic Diagnosis of Recurrences. Current State

The clinical utility of immunoscintigraphy for diagnosis of recurrences is a current subject of debate among physicians and surgeons in oncology and nuclear medicine specialists, some of whom are skeptical about the efficiency of the method, particularly its capacity for specific visualisation of all tumour sites. It is thus of interest to investigate the reasons for this skepticism - which is sometimes warranted, sometimes exaggerated - before considering the future prospects that should make this method of specific imaging more credible to most clinicians.

Methodological Heterogeneity

Immunoscintigraphysuffers perhaps first of all from a great methodological heterogeneity which can be interrupted as a lack of reliability. Several antibodies directed against different antigens have been used in clinical studies, though indeed those most often chosen have been anti-CEA antibodies. In addition to this difference in the nature of the antibodies selected, there has been uncertaintyas to the choice of form, whether intact antibodyor F(ab')2 or Fab' fragments. It has been generally agreed that the most suitable form for obtaining good contrast in the hours or days after injection is F(ab')2 fragments. Moreover, different antibodies in different forms have been labelled by different radionuclides. Iodine-131, used in the first clinical studies, has been replaced by iodine-123 and Indium-111 which possess characteristics that are clearly more favourable, providing greater accuracy and reproducibility of results. There is no doubt at the present time that antibodies should be labelled with technetium-99m in the future to facilitate use of all nuclear medicine centres. Labelling techniques with this radionuclide are not optimal at the present time and must be perfected before clinical validation is possible. Another limitation of immunoscintigraphyis the production of human anti-mouse antibodies which prevent repetition of an immunoscintigraphicexamination in the same patient.

Difficulties of Image Interpretation

Tumour contrast is often moderate, and count figures are not optimal with the radionuclide activities used (except for technetium-99m). To obtain reproducible results for several observers, images should be acquired in the best technical conditions and, if possible, in ECT mode. One problem in interpreting images is the lack of standardisation. With radionuclides such as indium-111 or technetium-99muptake is maximal in the liver and considerablygreater than in the tumour. To obtain interpretabletumour contrast, liver uptake must be "saturated" by lowering the upper threshold. Such image processing should be uniform to facilitate and standardize interpretationcriteria. In any event, image interpretationrequires solid experience and regular practice.

Clinical Results

When immunoscintigraphyis performed prospectivelyin the best technical conditions by a physician trained in interpreting such images, clinical results are quite satisfactory. With indium-111-labelled anti-CEA antibodies, diagnostic sensitivity and specificity are generally above 70% (5). The best results have been obtained for pelvic recurrences, with a sensitivity of over 80% for tumours larger than 1.5 cm. For the same pelvic sites, the accuracy of other imaging techniques is considerably lower, with diagnostic sensitivity below 50% (6). Immunoscintigraphic sensitivity is generally less good for abnormal tumour sites, particularly around the liver. Nor can liver metastases be visualised since radioantibody uptake is masked by high overall liver activity.

For the same anti-CEA antibodies labelled with iodine 123, clinical results are comparable to those of indium-111 for detection of pelvic recurrences with a similar population of patients (7). The advantage of iodine-123 is that liver metastases can be visualised since nonspecific hepatic activity is low, The major drawbacks are high cost and supply problems due to its relatively short half-life (13h).

The true clinical utility of this technique is determined by the percentage of cases in which recurrence is suspected because of a rise in serum CEA concentration, not confirmed by ultrasonography and computed tomography but clearly visualised by immunoscintigraphy. Curative surgery can then be performed, allowing significant improvement in patient survival. The percentage of such favourable cases, though difficult to determine exactly, is between 10 and 20% of patients explored by immunoscintigraphy. The short-term goal is to improve this percentage by better patient selection.

Future Prospects

Technological advances at short and middle term should improve the specificity of the method by reducing the number of false-positive results, make image interpretation easier and more accessible to all nuclear medicine departments and reduce the immunogenicity of injected radio-antibodies so that immunoscintigraphy can be repeated in the same patient.

Selection of New Antibodies

There is no cancer-specific antigen, particularly for gastrointestinal cancer, and it is unlikely that such an antigen exists. There is thus little likelihood of spectacular improvement in the oncologic specificity of antibodies, so that anti-CEA antibodies will probably remain the most suitable ones for imaging colorectal cancers.

New Methodological Approaches

Nonetheless, several new methodological approaches suggest that there will be marked improvement in image quality and thus greater facility in interpretation. First of all, the future of immunoscintigraphy depends on the use of technetium-99m for antibody labelling. With the injection activities (20 to 30 mCi), it will be possible to obtain satisfactory count figures and thus compensate in part for relatively poor tumour-to-normal tissue ratios. Current labelling methods have not yet been optimised, and their clinical validation must be confirmed. It is likely, if not certain, that within the next two years it will be possible to label F(ab')2 fragments of anti-CEA antibody with technetium-99m at a satisfactory in vitro and in vivo labelling stability.

One of the major current problems in image interpretation is nonspecific hepatic uptake which prevent visualisation of liver metastases and requires image processing for clear expression of tumour foci. It is thus essential to reduce this troublesome hepatic uptake. One promising method is in vivo labelling, which consists first in injecting a non-radiolabelled bispecific immunoconjugate with one site directed against the tumour antigen (e.g CEA) and one anti-hapten site. Two days after injection, when the immunoconjugate is taken up by tumour, the radioactive hapten is injected and diffuses rapidly towards the tumour where it is recognised by the anti-hapten site. Scintigraphy can be performed several hours after this second injection, which means that a short half-life radionuclide such as technetium-99m can be used. The first clinical studies have confirmed the expected reduction in nonspecific hepatic uptake (8). Another approach under study and experimentation in several laboratories is the use of metabolisable linkers which when introduced between antibody and chelate molecules, can serve as specific hepatic enzyme targets. The result is a radioantibody cleavage in the liver, with rapid urinary clearance of the chelate-radionuclide moiety. This theoretically attractive approach is still in the experimental stage and has not yet been clinically validated.

"Humanised Antibodies"

Another problem currently limiting the development of immunoscintigraphy is the production in patients of human anti-mouse antibodies (HAMA). This occurs in around 10-15% of patients after a first injection of F(ab')2 fragments of anti-CEA antibody. The presence of HAMA does not allow immunoscintigraphy to be repeated since the complexes formed after the second injection of antibodies prevent them from reaching their tumour target, thus giving false-negative results. It will be possible in the future to reduce the frequency of HAMA production by replacing murine antibodies with "humanised" antibodies in which only the specific binding site is of murine origin (the idiotypic site).

On the whole, immunoscintigraphyis a definitely useful imaging method for early detection of colorectal cancer recurrences, but it needs to be optimised before routine use in nuclear medicine departments is possible. In the future, this technique can be usefully extended to intraoperative detection of small tumour targets using a hand held probe for detection of radioactivity.

Radioimmunoguided Surgery

With the tumour-to-normal tissue ratios (between 5 and 10) obtained after injection of radiolabelled antibodies, it is theoretically possible to detect small superficial tumours less than a centimeter in diameter (9). This situation occurs during an operation when the surgeon can scan the abdominal cavity with a hand held probe to detect radioactivity. It is thus possible to resect small tumours which would not have been seen with the naked eye even of an experienced surgeon. This interesting detection method has been under experimentation for several years by Dr. Martin's team at the University of Ohio (10). The advantage of iodine-125, the radionuclide used, is that it emits low-energy gamma radiation. In these conditions, the probe only picks up the radiation emitted by the superficial tumour target, and there is no interference from nonspecific radiation originating in the underlying normal tissues since it is absorbed before reaching the detector. In a study of 32 patients with a suspected recurrence, radioimmunoguided surgery after injection of iodine-125-labelled antibodies allowed detection of a recurrence in 81% of patients. In 6 patients (18%), this technique was the only one to identify the recurrence site(s).

Unfortunately, in vivo use of iodine-125 is limited because of its long physical half-life. It is thus likely that the authorities in the different European countries which control the medical use of radionuclides will not approve routine injection of iodine-125-labelled antibodies. Recourse to other radionuclides with a shorter half-life will thus be necessary. Indium-111 and technetium-99m have a favourable physical half-life, but their gamma radiation energy is probably too strong and thus detrimental to depth resolution. The first clinical results with these two radionuclides are not as good as those obtained with iodine-125, thus confirming these limitations.

The future of radioimmunoguidedsurgery is therefore dependent on finding a radionuclide for antibody labelling which has a half-life of 2 to 8 days and emits low-energy radiation easily absorbed by a thin layer of tissue.

Conclusion

The true clinical utility of radiolabelled monoclonal antibodies can only be determined by the benefit that patients receive from their use, that is, by a significant improvement in their survival. Immunoscintigraphycomplemented by radioimmunoguidedsurgery can contribute to reaching this goal. In the still limited number of cases, immunoscintigraphyhas been the only method capable of early visualization of a recurrence totally resected by the surgeon. Radioimmunoguidedsurgery has also enabled complete excision of recurrences. However, the problems which remain must be resolved to allow these new diagnostic methods to be fully credible.

References

1. GoldenbergD.M. et al (1978) Use of radiolabelled antibodies to carcinoembryonicantigen for detection and localisation of diverse cancers by external photoscanning. New.Eng.J.Med.298;1384.

2. Martin D.T. et al (1985) Intraoperativeradioimmunodetectionof colorectal tumour with a hand-held radiation detector. Am.J.Surg.150; 672.

3. Martin E.W. et al (1980) Sixty second-look procedures indicated primarily by rise in serial carcinoembryonic antigen. J.Surg.Res. 28;389.

4. O'Dwyer P.J. et al (1988) Reoperation directed by carcinoembryonic antigen; the importance of a thorough preoperative evaluation. Am.J.Surg.155; 277.

5. ChetanneauA. et al (1989) Histological correlation of 17 prospective immunoscintigraphies of recurrences of colorectal carcinomas using Indium-111-labelled anti-CEA and/or 19-9 monoclonal antibodies. Eur.J.Nucl.Med. 15; 302.

6. Baum R.P. et al (1989) Special aspects of radioimmunoimaging of colon carcinoma. In "Immunotherapy and scintigraphy of tumours with monoclonal antibodies". A.A.Epenetos, E.Oberhausen, R.A. Reisfield, eds. W.Zuckschwerdt Verlag Munchen.pp.38-48.

7. Delaloye B. et al (1986) Detection of colorectal carcinoma by emission-computerised tomography after injection of I-123-labelled Fab or F(ab')2 fragments from monoclonal ant-carcinoembryonic antibodies. J.Clin.Invest. 77; 301.

8. Stickney D.R. et al (1990) Bifunctional antibody: ZCE/CHA 111-Indium BLEDTA-1V clinical imaging in colorectal carcinoma. Antib.Immunoconj.Radioph.3.

9. Rockoff S.D. et al (1990) Theoretical limitations in the immunodiagnostic imaging of cancer with computed tomography and nuclear scanning. Cancer Res.40; 3054.

10. Sardi A. et al (1989) Intra-abdominal recurrence of colorectal cancer detected by radioimmunoguided surgery (RIGS system). Arch.Surg. 124; 56.

USE OF 123-I RADIOLABELLED F(AB')2 FRAGMENTS OF ANTI-CEA MONOCLONAL ANTIBODY FOR THE DETECTION OF PRIMARY AND METASTATIC GASTROINTESTINAL CARCINOMAS

A.Bamias J.M.Sackier H.P.Kalofonos B.Dhokia D.Snook K.Bosslet C.Wood and A.A.Epenetos

Summary

F(ab')2 fragments of an anti-CEA monoclonal antibody were radiolabelled with 123-I and used to study eleven patients with various types of gastrointestinal carcinomas. The antibody scans detected primary or metastatic disease in 4 out of 7 patients with known disease and they suggested the existence of disease in 3 cases, in sites not detected by conventional techniques. In 1 patient, liver metastases were detected with the antibody scan 3 months earlier than with CT scan examination. Absence of disease was confirmed in 3 patients in complete remission. These results indicate that external scintigraphy using 123-I labelled F(ab')2 fragments of anti-CEA monoclonal antibodies may be a useful tool in monitoring patients with gastrointestinal tumours in terms of confirming the results of conventional methods or revealing disease sites undetected by conventional radiology.

R. P. Baum et al. (eds.), Clinical Use of Antibodies, 45–53.

Introduction

Radiolabelled anti-CEA antibodies have been used extensively for the detection of CEA expressing tumours. Many workers (10,13,4,1) have used polyclonal antibodies with promising results in some cases but the low immunoreactivity or specificity of these antibodies was a serious drawback. The production of monoclonal antibodies (12) resulted in a new interest in the use of CEA specific antibodies and initial results were encouraging (14). However, there are still serious problems caused by the low absolute amount of antibody reaching the target, the non specific uptake of the antibodies, the formation of immune complexes and degradation of the immunoconjugates (17) as well as the high levels of blood pool radioactivity. Several approaches were used in order to minimize the above limitations including the use of F(ab')2 and Fab fragments (6,18) or single photon emission computerised tomography (14).

Aim

In this study we report our experience on the immunolocalisation of gastrointestinal tumours and especially liver metastases using F(ab')2 fragments of anti-CEA monoclonal antibody labelled with 123-I.

Patients and Methods

Eleven patients, aged 30-70 years (mean 56 years) with various gastrointestinal carcinomas (Table 1) were studied. All patients gave their written informed consent prior to entering this study.

Monoclonal antibody: BW431/26 anti-CEA monoclonal antibody (Behringwerke) was used. Each patient received an intravenous injection and the average amount of the administered protein was 500 μgrs (250-700 μgrs).

Iodination: The antibodies were iodinated with 123-I (AERE Harwell) using the N-Bromosuccinimidemethod (16). Free iodine was removed by gel filtration using Sephadex G50 column and eluted with phosphate buffered saline (PBS,pH 7.4) under sterile conditions and millipore filtered prior to administration. The radioactivity scans were performed at ten minutes, 24 hours and 48 hours after the administrationof the labelled antibody using a 40cm field-of-view gamma camera with a medium energy collimator.

Results

The antibodies used in the study were radiolabelled to a specific activity of 4-7mCi/mgr. The final solution contained more than 95% of the total amount of the radioiodine used for the iodination.

Table 1 summarises the histological diagnoses and the antibodies administered to each patient and compares the findings of conventional investigation (biochemical, X-ray, CT scan, ultrasound, technetium 99m colloidal scan) with those of antibody-guided scanning.

Primary or metastatic disease was revealed in 4 out of 7 cases (sensitivity 57%) (Fig.1. There were no false positive scans (specificity 100%). In 3 patients in complete remission the antibody scans confirmed the absence of disease. In 3 cases radioimmunoscintigraphyrevealed possible disease sites not detected with the conventional investigation. In one of these cases the antibody scan showed a focal area of increased antibody uptake in the liver, while the CT scan and ultrasound examination were negative. Liver involvement was confirmed by CT scan 3 months after the antibody scan. In the second patient gastric infiltration, shown by the antibody scan, was confirmed later by gastroscopy (Fig.1) while in the third case the findings of the antibody were not confirmed by further investigation due to rapid deterioration of the patient.

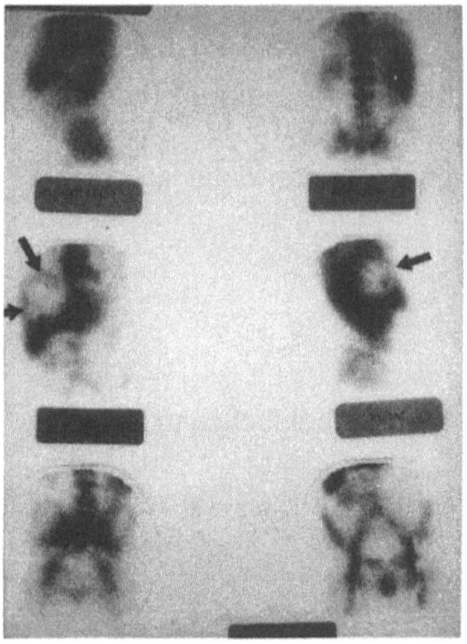

Fig.1.

a) Cold area in the liver (arrows) at 10 minutes after antibody injection in a patient with colon adenocarcinoma.

b) Increased uptake in the same area at 24 hours. There is also increased radioactivity in the stomach (arrows). Gastroscopy performed after the antibody scan confirmed gastric infiltration not detected by conventional radiology examination.

Discussion

Gastrointestinal carcinomas usually express CEA very intensely and may show high CEA serum levels as demonstrated by anti-CEA antibodies (7). The circulating CEA does not appear to influence anti-CEA antibodies localisation in the tumour when they are administered to patients with gastrointestinal carcinomas (14). Intravenous administration of such monoclonal antibodies has been used by many to detect primary or metastatic CEA expressing tumours (3,6). The results of this study indicate that 123-I radiolabelled F(ab')2 fragments of anti-CEA monoclonal antibodies can produce successful imaging of primary of metastatic lesions by external body scintigraphy in patients with gastrointestinal tumours. Furthermore, in several cases antibody scans detected lesions not revealed by conventional methods. Therefore, they could be of value during the follow-up of these patients. Both F(ab')2 and Fab fragments have been used instead of intact antibodies because of their different kinetics and metabolism which seem to be preferable for immunoscintigraphy(6,11). Non specific uptake of F(ab')2 fragments is less than that of intact antibody and their clearance from the circulation is more rapid. In addition, the rate of immune immunoscintigraphic studies taking into consideration that Fab fragmented binding to tumour is less than F(ab')2 and intact antibody (6). Immunoscintigraphy after F(ab')2 anti-CEA monoclonal antibody administration can detect liver metastases, which is the most common metastatic site and one of the most frequent causes of death in patients with gastrointestinal carcinoma. Nevertheless, liver involvement was not detected in 3 cases. In fact, in the first 24 hours liver metastases are demonstrated as cold areas which, in the positive cases, are filled in progressively. This is probably due to alterations in the circulation caused by the metastatic disease. Since the short half life of 123-I make late imaging impossible, it seems that in certain cases 48 hours are not enough for the accumulation of the antibody in the involved areas. 111-In may overcome the problem of short half life and in fact it has already been used for imaging gastrointestinal tumours (17). Recently, new methods of labelling monoclonal antibodies with 99mTc have been developed (9). These methods can provide radiolabelled antibodies with enhanced in vivo stability and therefore promising clinical utility.

TABLE 1

Case	Age (years)	Histology	Antibody	Findings of antibody scans	Findings of conventional method
1	48	Colon adeno carcinoma	$F(ab')_2$	a) Cold area in the right lobe of the liver in the first scan while increasing accumulation of activity was observed in the periphery of this area. At 24 hours increased uptake in the same area. b) Increased uptake in the mucosa of the stomach.	Liver metastases in the right lobe of the liver with CT scan.
2	70	Colon adeno-carcinoma	intact	No evidence of disease	No disease
3	50	Rectal adeno-carcinoma	$F(ab')_2$	Focal cold area in the liver in the first scan without later accumulation.	Liver metastases in CT scan
4	65	Gastric adeno-carcinoma	F(ab')2	a) Focal areas of increased uptake at the mediastinum at 24 and 48 hrs scans b) Focal area below the heart and at the region of lower cervical nodes or thoracic inlet at 24 and 48 hrs scans. c) Increased activity along the stomach at 24 and 48 hrs scans. d) Focal areas in the region of epi-gastrium inferior to the stomach possibly representing uptake of the paraortic nodes.	No evidence of disease in X-rays
5	36	Fibrolamellar hepatoma	intact	No evidence of disease.	No evidence of disease with CT scan

6	48	Colon adeno-carcinoma	intact	No evidence of disease	a) Metastases in the lungs with CT scan b) Paraortic nodes involvement detected with CT scan c) Possible liver metastases with CT scan
7	52	Pancreatic carcinoma	F(ab')2	a) Two focal areas of increased uptake in the right lobe of the liver b) Diffuse area of increased activity in the epigastrium extending to the mid-abdomen. c) Focal activity in the pelvis adjacent to the region of rectum or sacrum at 24 hrs scan.	a) Liver metastases in CT scan b) Large pancreatic tumour in CT scan
8	63	Colon adeno-carcinoma	$F(ab')_2$	a) Defects in the liver centrally and in the upper right and left lobes.	a) Liver metastases in the right and left lobe of the liver in CT scan.
9	58	Rectal adeno-carcinoma	F(ab')2	Focal areaof increased uptake in the central liver at 24 and 48 hrs.	a) CT scan 3 months after the antibody scan confirmed the liver involvement.
10	41	Rectal adeno-carcinoma	intact	No evidence of disease.	Clinical evaluation suggested complete remission.
11	61	Gastric adeno-carcinoma	intact	Diffuse increase of activity in the liver without any focal uptake.	Well defined areas in both right and left lobes of the liver in colloidal scan.

Finally, the route of administrationis another factor which is also worth studying. Regional antibody administration has already been used by many investigators (8,15) for therapy rather than imaging. Antibody administration through the hepatic artery could be useful in the detection of liver metastases and in fact it has been used in order to achieve a better accumulation in the liver (5). This method seems to be promising in therapy for liver metastases (Pawlikowska et al,1986) but intravenous administration is more simple and therefore more applicable for diagnostic purposes.

In conclusion, this study demonstratesthat 123-I labelled F(ab')2 fragmentsof an anti-CEA monoclonal antibodycan successfullylocalise gastrointestinaltumours and may be a useful tool in staging and monitoring patients.

References

1) Begent R.H.K. et al (1980) Radioimmunolocalisationof tumours by external scintigraphy after administration of 131-I antibody to human chronic gonadotropin: preliminary communication. J.Royl.Soc.Med. 73:624-630

2) Berche C. et al(1982) Tomoscintigraphyfor detectinggastrointestinaland medullary thyroid cancers: first clinical results using radiolabelled monoclonal antibodies against carcino embryonic antigen. Br.Med.J. 285: 1447-1451

3) Chatal J.F. et al (1984) Immunoscintigraphyof colon carcinoma. J.Nucl.Med. 25: 307-314

4) Dykes D.W. et al (1980) Localisationof tumour deposits by externalscanningafter injection of radiolabelled anti-carcinoembryonicantigen Br.Med.J. 280: 220-222

5) Delaloye B. et al (1985) First approach to therapy of liver metastases in colorectal carcinoma by intrahepatically infused 131-I labelled monoclonal anti-CEA antibodies. Eur.J.Nucl.Med.11:A37

6) Delaloye B et al (1986) Detection of colorectal carcinoma by emission computerised tomography after injection of 123-I labelled Fab and F(ab')2 fragments from monoclonal anti-carcinoembryonicantigen antibodies. J.Clin.Inv. 77: 301-311

7) Endo T. et al (1985) Immunohistologicdistribution of CEA defined by human anti-CEA antibody in the serum of a colonic cancer patient.Cancer56: 2205-2211

8) Epenetos A.A, et al (1984) Antibody guided irradiation of malignant lesions. Lancet 1:1441-1443

9) Fritzberg A.R. et al (1988) Specific and stable labelling of antibodies with technetium-99m with a diamide dithiolate chelating agent. Proc.Natl.Acad.Sci.USA85: 4025-4029

10) Goldenberg D. et al (1978) Use of radiolabelled antibodies to carcinoembryonic antigen for the detection and localisation of diverse cancers by external photoscanning. New Engl.J.Med. 298: 1384-1388

11) Kalofonos H.P. et al (1988) Kinetics, quantitative analysis and radioimmunolocalisation using indium-111 HMFG1 monoclonal antibody in patients with breast cancer.Br.J.Cancer59: 934-942

12) Kohler G and Milstein C (1975) Continuous culture of fused cells secreting antibody of predefined specificity. Nature 256: 465-467

13) Mach J.P et al (1980) Tumour localisation of radiolabelled antibodies against carcinoembryonic antigen in patients with carcinoma. New Engl.J.Med. 305: 5-10

14) Mach J.P. et al (1981) Use of 131-I radiolabelled monoclonal anti-CEA antibodies for the detection of human carcinomas by external photoscanning and tomoscintigraphy.Immunology Today 2: 239-249

15) Pectasides D. et al (1986) Antibody guided irradiation of malignant pleural and pericardial effusions.Br.J.Cancer53: 727-732

16) Reay P. (1982) Use of N-bromosuccinimide for the iodination of proteins for radioimmunoassay. Ann.Clin.Biochem. 19: 129-133

17) Riva P et al (1988) Antibody-guided diagnosis an Italian experience on CEA-expressing tumours In.J.Cancer Supplement 2: 114-120

18) Siccardi A.G. et al (1989) Immunoscintigraphy of adenocarcinomas by means of radiolabelled F(ab')2 fragments of an anti-carcinoembryonic antigen monoclonal antibody: a multicentre study. Cancer Res. 49: 3095-3103.

BISPECIFIC MONOCLONAL ANTIBODIES FOR TWO PHASE RADIOIMMUNOTHERAPY

K. Bosslet , A. Steinstraesser ,P. Hermentin , L. Kuhlmann , A. Bruynck , M. Magerstaedt , G. Seemann , A. Schwarz and H.H. Sedlacek

Abstract

Starting from the moderate therapeutic effects of MAb guided radioimmunotherapyin the treatment of carcinomas, we presented a two phase radioimmunotherapy concept based on bispecific MAbs which might be more effective. To work out this concept we first showed that penetration into human carcinoma xenografts as well as long term storage of intact MAb outside the carcinoma cells are possible. Epitope saturation was however not yet obtained despite the large MAb doses injected i.v for 10 days. Second we generated hybridomas producing high avidity anti metal chelate MAbs (anti DTPY-Y). These hybridomas were fused with hybridomas producing MAbs selective for CEA or GIT-mucin, and stable bispecific MAb producing quadromas were obtained. THE purification of these bispecific anti Cea x anti DTPA-Y or anti GIT-mucin x anti DTPA-Y MAbs, their detailed molecular characterization and potential value we are going to work out.

Introduction

Immunoscintigraphy using Tc-99m-labelled MAbs (34) is going to become a routine diagnostic method for the specific in vivo detection of tumors (3,4,25,26) or inflammatory processes (21,21,22,5)

In contrast, radioimmunotherapyusing MAbs tagged with I-131 or Y-90 has not yet been accepted in oncology as a treatment modality despite a few encouraging early reports (14,13). This is mainly due to the small amounts of radiolabelled Mabs bound to the tumor site and the unfavourable whole body distribution and metabolisation of intact immunoglobulins or their

R. P. Baum et al. (eds.), Clinical Use of Antibodies, 55–68.

fragments (37). If a radioactive α- or β-emitter or a toxic drug is directly coupled to the MAb or its fragment the above mentioned unfavourable whole body distribution would bring much harm to many non tumor tissues especially bone marrow.

It may be possible to circumvent these problems using one of the recently suggested two phase approaches (1,2,16,17,32,12). These approaches assume a long term non toxic targeting phase of a modified MAb and a second short term toxic binding or activation phase of a small hydrophilic molecule.

In this report we show that it is possible to target significant amounts of MAb to human colon carcinoma xenografts and to store the MAb for many days at the tumor site. If such a MAb would have two arms with different specificities, one against the tumor, the second against a small hydrophilic metal chelate it should be possible to target a quickly - distributing and penetrating chelate very efficiently to the tumor. Because of its short plasma half life and its complete extracellular distribution, a molecule like DTPA-Y90 should bring little harm to the normal tissue but would hopefully be retained at the anti DTPA arm of the bispecific MAb.

Furthermore this paper presents our efforts to generate bispecific anti tumor x anti DTPA-Y90 MAbs to be able to optimize the condition for the concept of two phase radioimmunotherapy.

Material and Methods

Immunohistochemical investigations

Thin sections (6 μm) from cryopreserved human tumor xenografts were investigated using the highly sensitive APAAP-technique (Cordell et al. 1984) without any fixation.

Percolation and saturation studies

Human colon carcinoma (CoCa4) bearing nude mice (three animals/group) were 10x injected i.v. with 250 μg each of Mabs BW 431, BW 494 or BW 227 (6,7) for ten consecutive days. Tumors were resected at various days after stop of i.v. injection and processed for immunohistochemical investigations.

Production of DTPA specific MAb

As immunogen, 19 moles of SCN-benzyl-DTPA were coupled to 1 mole of human serum albumen (HSA-benzyl-DTPA)(10). Immunogen was incubated with a 100 fold molar excess of Y-89 for 2 hrs at R.T. to saturate DTPA with Y. Free Y was removed by Sephadex G-25 column chromatography. Groups of 5 Balb/c mice were injected s.c. at day 0 with 25 μg of HSA-benzyl-DTPA-Y complex mixed with an equal amount of complete Freunds adjuvant (CFA). At days 7 and 14 the animals received the same dose of immunogen admixed to incomplete Freunds adjuvant (IFA). One week later at day 21 immunogen was diluted in PBS and given i.p. Fusion was performed at day 37 (23) using the SP20/Ag4 myeloma cells (33) as a fusion partner.

Screening of hybridomas

Hybridoma supernatants were screened for the presence of anti HSA-benzyl-DTPA-Y MAb using an ELISA system in which the immunogen was attached to the solid phase (50 ng/well) of round bottom polystyrol microtiter plates (Fa. Nunc). Bound MAb was detected using an alkaline phosphatase labelled goat anti mouse Ig antibody combined with the alcohol dehydrogenase-diaphorase amplification system (35).

MAb purification

Hybridomas were cultured in serum free Iscoves medium and MAb was purified from the supernatants according to (15).

Competition ELISA

Purified MAb was incubated with increasing concentrations of DTPA-Y or other chelates for 1 hr at R.T.. These mixtures were added to solid phase attached HSA-benzyl-DTPA-Y in percoated round bottom polystyrol plates and the efficiency of MAb chelete interaction was calculated by the molar excess of chelate leading to 50 % binding inhibition to the solid phase attached immunogen (IC_{50} value).

Introduction of genetic markers

Deficiency of HGPRT ($HGPRT^-$) was introduced in the $HGPRT^+$ hybridomas 431 and 494 by culturing the hybridomas for several weeks in increasing concentrations of TG. HAT sensitivity was obtained at 100 μg TG/ml for hybridoma 431 and 494. Deficiency for TK (TK^-) was introduced in the TK^+ hybridoma 2050/174 by culturing the hybridoma for several weeks in increasing concentrations of BrdU. HAT sensitivity was obtained at 1000 μg BrdU/ml.

Quadroma production

Hybridomas 431 and 494 carrying the HGPRT⁻ marker were fused each with the hybridoma 2050/174 carrying the TK⁻ marker at a 1:1 ratio. Outgrowing quadromas were selected in HAT medium.

ELISA for detection of bispecific MAb

To each individual well of polystyrol round bottom plate coated with 50 ng HSA-benzyl-DTPA-Y per well, 50 μl of quadroma supernatant was added and incubated for 30' at R.T.. After 3x washing, 50 μl of biotinylated anti-idiotypic MAb selective for MAb BW 431 (MAb BW 2064) or 50 μl of biotinylated MAb selective for MAb 494 (MAb BW 705) (9) was added. After washing the amount of solid phase bound bispecific MAb was visualized using the avidin-biotin peroxidase system (Vector, Burlingname).

Results

Percolation and storage of i.v. injected anti CEA and anti GIT mucin MAbs in human colon carcinoma xenografts.

Groups of nude mice carrying the CoCa4 human tumor xenograft received 10 high dose MAb infusions as described in Material and Methods. Immunohistochemical investigations revealed that MAb BW 431 selective for CEA as well as MAb BW 494 binding to stomach, pancreas and colon carcinoma associated GIT-mucin (6,7) could penetrate and bind to the colon carcinoma tissue (Fig.1, data shown for MAb BW 494). At the end of the injection period at day 10 MAb BW 494 could be visualized very efficiently using a rabbit anti mouse IgG_1 second antibody (Fig.1a). The MAb was located at the tumor cell membrane, in the lumen and in the interstitial space. A very similar observation was made at day 20 (Fig.1b) or at day 30 (Fig.1c) indicating that the MAb BW 494 once penetrated into the tumor, remaining there for a long period of time. MAb BW 227, selective for a mycoplasma associated epitope, did not bind to the tumor tissue at neither point investigated (Fig.1d). Addition of MAb BW 494 to CoCa4 tissue sections followed by the anti mouse IgG_1 second antibody resulted in a staining reaction only marginally stronger than the second antibody incubation (Fig.1e), indicating that the long term i.v. injection allowed MAb BW 494 to bind to the majority of accessible epitopes.

To investigate, whether the high dose and long term i.v. injection had saturated all epitopes an isotype switch variant detection experiment was done. CoCa4 tissue sections from i.v. treated animals were incubated with MAb BW 494 IgG_{2a} selective second antibody system. An essentially identical staining reaction was seen (Fig.1f) indicating that epitope saturation was not obtained despite the high dose and long term i.v. injection of MAb BW 494. Essentially identical data were received using the CEA specific MAb BW 431 indicating that penetration and long term storage of MAbs in human carcinoma xenografts seem to be principally possible.

Generation of anti DTPA-Y MAbs

After having realised that penetration and long term storage of intact Mabs is possible in human tumor xenografts, we decided to produce bispecific antitumor x anti DTPA-Y. Because no high affinity anti DTPA-Y Mabs were available (30), we started to generate these MAbs ourselves. As immunogen HSA-benzyl-DTPA-Y was used a direct binding ELISA on HSA-benzyl-DTPA-Y solid phase or a competition ELISA. The individual MAbs showed different strength of binding to the various chelates. In contrast to our expectation DTPA-Y was not the best inhibitor. Out of the Y chelates investigated the EDTA-Y was the best inhibitor. But some MAbs were also efficiently inhibited using uncomplexed DTPA or EDTA or their complexes formed with irrelevant ions. Structurally related substances like diaminoethan or transaconitic acid had no significant inhibitory effect indicating that the MAb chelate binding is not simply due to charge or hydrophobic interactions, but seems to be more complex. Out of the five MAbs presented in table 1 MAb BW 2050/174 was elected for further use because of its very efficient binding to EDTA-Y and its still reasonable binding to DTPA-Y.

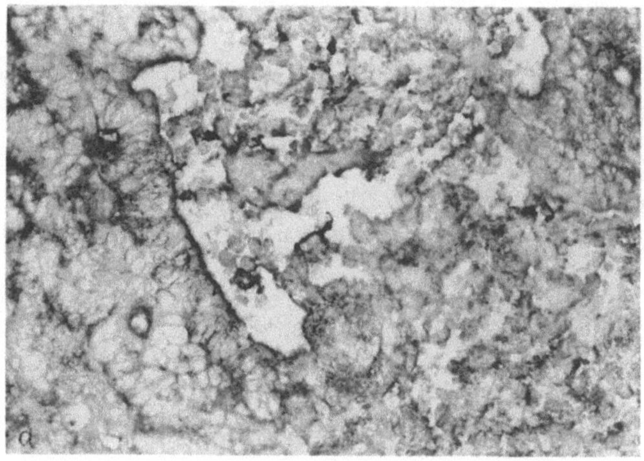

Fig 1a

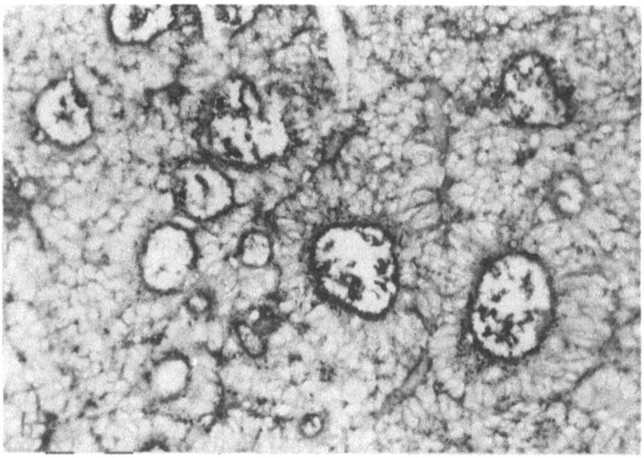

Fig.1b

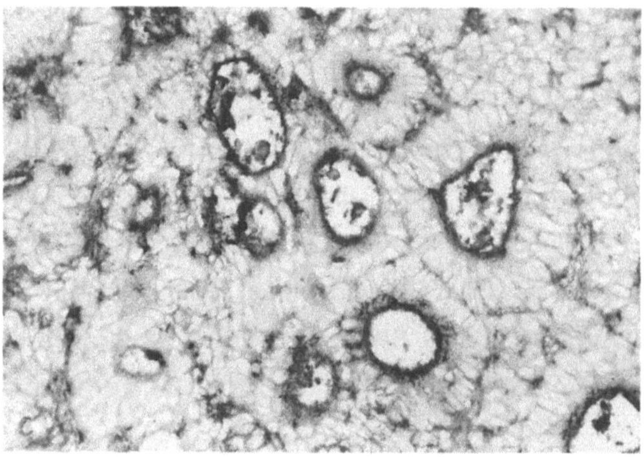

Fig.1c

Figs 1a - c *Represents tissue from MAb BW 494 treated mice removed at days 10,20 or 30 respectively and stained using a goat anti mouse* IgG_1 *second antibody*

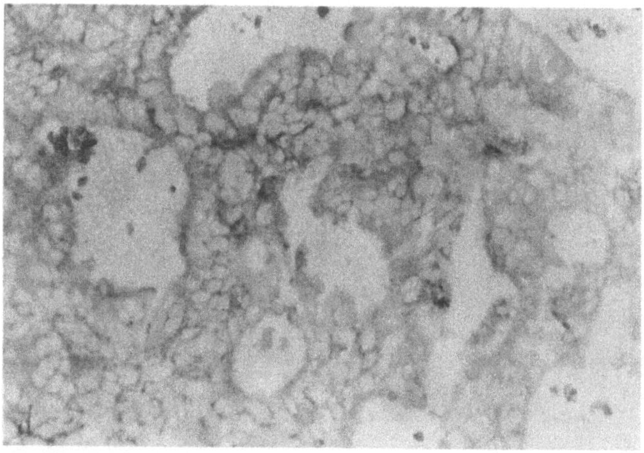

Fig. 1d *Represents tissue from MAb BW 227 treated mice removed at day 20 and stained as described above*

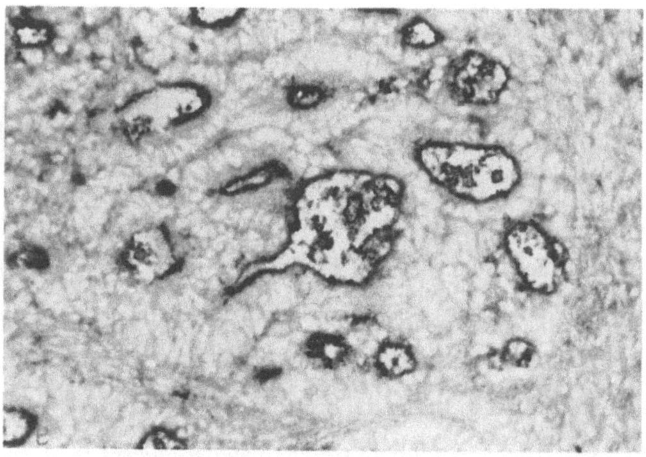

Fig.1e *Represents tissue from Mab BW 494 treated mice removed at day 30 and stained by addition of 20 μg/ml MAb BW 494 followed by a goat anti mouse* IgG_1 *second antibody*

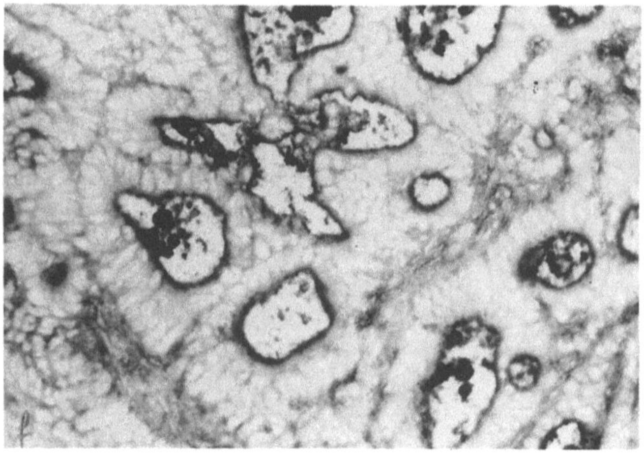

Fig.1f *Represents tissue from mice treated as in Fig.1e. Staining was by addition of 20 μg/ml of MAb BW 494 IgG_{2a} followed by a goat anti mouse IgG_{2a} second antibody*

Construction of bispecific MAbs

As tumor specific MAbs MAb BW 431 selective for CEA (7) and MAb BW 494 selective for the GIT-mucin (6) were chosen. In clinical trials the potential of both MAbs to localize colorectal stomach and pancreas carcinomas in patients was proven. The hybridomas 431 and 494 were selected for HGPRT deficiency and fused each with hybridoma 2050/174 selected for TK deficiency (see Materials and Methods). The arising quadromas were selected in HAT medium and screened for the presence of bispecific MAb using a specifically developed antigen-antiidiotype ELISA system (see Materials and Methods). A typical fusion experiment was generated between 20 to 40 quadromas. Quadromas producing significant amounts (1 - 5 μg) of bispecific MAb were stabilised by 3x repetitive limiting dilution cloning. Stable quadromas were mass-cultured and procedures to purify the bispecific MAbs are presently worked out to separate the bispecific MAb from 9 potentially contaminated irrelevant MAb species present in quadroma supernatants (27).

Discussion

The present report introduces a two phase radioimmunotherapy approach which consists of essentially three steps:

1. A nontoxic tumor tissue penetration, binding and storage phase of a bispecific anti CEA x anti DTPA-Y (or anti GIT-mucin x anti DTPA-Y) MAb;

2. A waiting period of several days in which the nonspecifically bound bispecific MAb is eliminated from the body or metabolised in the liver parenchymal cells whereas the tumor bound MAb remains located extracellularly in the interstitial spaces or on the tumor cell membrane;

3. A short term binding phase of the radiolabelled DTPA-Y to the new receptor created on the tumor by the anti DTPA-Y arm of the bispecific MAb. Non bound DTPA-Y distributes extracellularly and is eliminated during a few minutes via the kidneys.

The experimental data generated support the assumptions made in the first step. It seems to be possible to get a significant tissue penetration of solid human carcinoma xenografts after repetitive i.v. injection for 10 days of high doses of tumor specific MAb. This finding is in contrast to the reports of others who show that single i.v. injection of radiolabelled MAb leads to the rim of the tumor only (38,29) as revealed using autoradiography. The immunohistochemical methodology applied in our work allowed an exact localization of the MAb at the tumor cell membranes, the interstitial space and the lumen, i.e outside the tumor cells. THis localization was observed at the stop of i.v. therapy at day 10 (Fig 1a) as well as on day 20 (Fig. 1b) and on day 30 (Fig. 1c). This tissue penetration and long term storage phase was shown to be similar for two individual MAbs, the CEA-specific MAb BW 431 and the GIT-mucin specific MAb BW 494 (6,7). Despite of the repetitive injection of high doses of MAb for 10 days (corresponding to 8 g of MAb/patient) no epitope saturation in the tumor tissue was obtained yet (Fig. 1f). Tissue penetration could be optimised in future trials using MAb fragments or genetically engineered domain antibodies (18,39).

The second step of our two phase radioimmunotherapy approach was experimentally proven by Steinstraesser et al (36) who showed that biosynthetically as well as In-111-labelled MAb is metabolised in the liver parenchymal cells, i.e. no more accessible from outside.

The efficiency of the third step to get a strong binding of the Y-labelled chelate to the anti-chelate arm of the bispecific MAb is certainly depending on the efficiency of the anti-chelate arm to the chelate metal complex. Therefore we tried to generate high affinity anti DTPA-Y MAbs by immunizing Balb/c mice with an especially synthesised highly immunogenic hapten carrier complex. The immunization with this HSA-benzyl-DTPA-Y complex resulted in the generation of 350 clones producing MAbs binding to the immunogen. Out of these MAbs those were elected which could be inhibited in their binding to the immunogen by free DTPA-Y or related compounds (Table I). Out of these hybridomas MAb BW 2050/174 was elected because its strong binding to DTPA-Y and its excellent binding to EDTA-Y. Why a MAb could be generated which binds more efficiently to EDTA-Y than to DTPA-Y despite the fact that the HSA-benzyl-DTPA-Y was used as immunogen can not be explained at the moment. Interestingly, all MAbs binding to DTPA-Y or EDTA-Y consisted of IgG_1 heavy chain and a -light chain. This is in contrast to all other MAbs generated by the authors in the Balb/c system which exclusively use a -light chain. The future has to show, whether the affinity of the single anti CEA or anti GIT-mucin arms of the quadroma produced bispecific MAbs is strong enough to keep these reagents attached to the tumor as long and as efficiently as the bivalent MAbs do. The most critical point in our approach is probably the affinity of the anti DTPA-Y arm to the free DTPA-Y or EDTA-Y which has to bind very efficiently in vivo to the new chelate specific receptor on the tumor created by the anti DTPA-Y arm of the bispecific MAb. The small hydrophilic DTPA-Y should be trapped by the anti DTPA-Y arm like a small hormone (31,24) by its receptor and should lead to a quick and efficient localization of the tumor.

At the moment it can not yet be decided which of the chelates (EDTA or benzyl-DTPA or DTPA, Table I) might be the best for in vivo applications. But the β-emitting isotope (Y-90) which can be very stably complexed to all of the three chelates (30) might be able to circumvent the problems of tumor heterogeneity and limited percolation (19,9) in human tissues due to its long range radiation (9 mm). We hope that the work described in this report might be the right way for the development of a new and more effective radioimmunotherapy of carcinomas.

Abbreviations used

CEA = carcinoembryonic antigen; GIT-mucin = gastrointestinal tract mucin; MAb = monoclonal antibody; SCN-benzylDTPA = isothiocyanatobenzyldiethylenetriaminepentaacetic acid; HSA = human serum albumen; PBS = phosphate buffered saline; R.T. = room temperature; HGPRT = hypoxanthine guanine phosphoribosyl transferase; TK = thymidine kinase; TG = thioguanine; BrdU = bromodeoxyuridine; HAT hypoxanthine aminopterin thymidine.

Acknowledgement

The technical assistance of C .Wetzler, K .Waldinger, H .Lind and N. Döring as well as the secretarial assistance of S. Lehnert are greatly appreciated.

References

1. Bagshaw KD (1987) Antibody directed enzymes revive anti-cancer prodrugs concept. Br J Cancer 56:531-540

2. Bagshaw KD, Spinger CJ, Searle F (1988) A cytotoxic agent can be generated selectively at cancer sites. Br J Cancer 58:700-704

3. Baum RP, Hottenrott LC, Schwarz A, Hör G (1988) Immunoscintigraphyof known and occult metastatic colorectal carcinoma with Tc-99m anti CEA monoclonal antibody. J Nucl Med 28:834

4. Baum RP, Hertel A, Lorenz M, Schwarz A, Encke A, Hör G (1989) Tc-99m labelled anti CEA monoclonal antibody for tumor immunoscintigraphy. First clinical results. Nucl Med Commun 10:345-352

5. Becker W, Borst U, Fischbach W, Pasarka B, Schäfer R, Börner W, (1989) Kinetic data of in-vivo labelled granulocytes in humans with a murine Tc-99m-labelled monoclonal antibody. Eur J Nucl Med 15:361-366

6. Bosslet K, Kern HF, Kanzy EJ, Steinstraesser A, Schwarz A, Lüben G, Schorlemmer HU, Sedlacek HH (1986) A monoclonal antibody with binding and inhibiting activity towards human pancreatic carcinoma cells. Cancer Immunol Immunother 23:185-191

7. Bosslet K, Steinstraesser A, Schwarz A, Harthus HP, Lüben G, Kuhlmann L, Sedlacek HH (1988a) Quantitative considerations supporting the irrelevance of circulating serum CEA for the immunoscintigraphic visualization of CEA expressing carcinomas. Eur J Nucl Med 14:523-528

8. Bosslet K, Döring N, Seeman G, Schultz G, Sedlacek HH (1988b) Immunological tailoring of monoclonal antibodies for immunotherapy of pancreatic carcinoma. Int J Cancer Suppl 2:25-88

9. Bosslet K, Keweloh HCh, Hermentin P, Muhrer KH, Sedlacek HH, Schulz G (1990) Percolation and binding of monoclonal antibody BW 494 to pancreatic carcinoma tissues during high dose immunotherapy and consequences for future therapy modalities. Br J

Cancer 61:Suppl in press

10. Brechbiel MW, Gansow OA, Atcher RW, Colcher D, Schlom J, Esteban J, Simpson DE (1986) Synthesis of 1-(p-isothiocyanatobenzyl)derivative of DTPA and EDTA. Antibody labeling and tumor-imaging studies. Inorganic Chem 25:2772-2781

11. Cordell JL, Falini B, Erber WN, Gash AK, Abdulaziz Z, Macdonald S, Pulford KAF, Stein H, Mason DY (1984) Immunoenzymatic labeling of monoclonal antibodies using immune complexes of alkaline phosphatase and monoclonal antialkaline phosphatase. J Histochem Cytochem 32:219-224

12. Doussal JM Le, Martin M, Gautherat E, Delaage M, Barbet M (1989) In vitro and in vivo targeting of radiolabelled monovalent and divalent haptens with dual specificity monoclonal antibody conjugates: Enhanced divalent hapten affinity for cell bound antibody conjugates. J Nucl Med 30 : 1358-1366

13. Epenetos AA, (1987) Phase I clinical trial of intraperitoneally administered radiolabelled monoclonal antibodies in the treatment of advanced ovarian cancer. In: New tumour markers and their monoclonal antibodies. Edit. by R. Klapdor, pp 521-530, Stuttgart: Thieme, 1987

14. Epenetos AA and Kosmas C (1989) Monoclonal antibodies for imaging and therapy. Br J Cancer 59:153-155

15. Ey PL, Prowse SJ, Jenkin CR (1978) Isolation of pure IgG_1, IgG_{2a}, IgG_{2b} immunoglobulins from mouse serum using protein A-sepharose. Immunochemistry 15:429-436

16. Hnatowich DJ, Virzi F, Rusckowski M (1987) Investigations of avidin and biotin for imaging applications. J Nucl Med 28:1294-1302

17. Hnatowich DJ, Rowlinson G, Ruskowski M, Snook D, Epenetos AA (1989) Tumour localisation studies with streptavidin and biotin. Br J Cancer 59:308

18. Huse WD, Sastry L, Iverson SA, Kang AS, Alting-Mees M, Burton DR, Benkovic SJ, Lerner RA (1989) Generation of large combinatorial library of the immunoglobulin repertoire in phage lambda. Science 246:1275-1281

19. Jain KR, (1987) Transport of molecules in the tumour interstitium: A review. Cancer Res 47:3030-3061

20. Joseph K, Höffken H, Damann V (1987) In vivo labelling of granulocytes using ^{99m}Tc-labelled monoclonal antibodies: First clinical results. Nuc Compact 18:223-229

21. Joseph K, Höffken H, Bosslet K, Schorlemmer HU (1988a) Imaging of inflammation with granulocytes labelled in vivo. Nucl Med Commun 9:763-769

22. Josepk K, Höffken H, Bosslet K, Schorlemmer HU (1988b) In vivo labelling of granulocytes with ^{99m}Tc-anti-NCA monoclonal antibodies for imaging inflammation. Eur J Nucl Med

14:367-373

23. Köhler G, Milstein C (1975) Continuous cultures of fused cells secreting antibody of predefined specificity. Nature 256:495-496

24. Krenning EP, Breeman WAP, Kooij PPM, Lamaris JS, Bakkers WH, Koper JW, Ausema L, Reubi JC, Lamberts SWJ (1989) Localisation of endocrine-related tumours with radioiodinated analogue of somatostatin. The Lancet Febr. 4:242-244

25. Kroiss A, Tuchmann A, Schüller J, Weiss W, Wirth M, Auinger Ch, Neumayr A (1989) Tumor localization by immunoscintigraphy with anti-CEA antibody (Tc-99m MAk BW 431/26). Wiener klin Wschr 101:621-626

26. Lind P, Langsteger W, Költringer P, Lechner P, Beham A, Adrian-Schad K, Eber O (1989) ^{99m}Tc-labelled monoclonal anti-carcinoembryonicantigen antibody (BW 431/26). Scand I Gastroenterol 24:1205-1211

27. Milstein C, Cuello AC (1983) Hybrid hybridomas and their use in immunohistochemistry. Nature 305:537-540

28. Ong GL, Mathe MJ (1989) Penetration and binding of antibodies in experimental human solid tumors grown in mice. Cancer Res 49:4264-4273

29. Pervez S, Epenetos AA, Mooi WJ, Evans DJ, Rowlinson G, Dhokia B, Krausz T (1988) Localization of monoclonal antibody AUAI and its $F(ab')_2$ fragments in human tumour xenografts: an autoradiographic and immunohistochemical study. Int J Cancer Supp. 3:23-29

30. Rearden DT, Meares CF, Goodwin DA, McTigue M, David GS, Stone MR, Leung JP, Bartholomew RM, Frincke JM (1985) Antibodies against metal chelates. Nature 316:265-268

31. Reubi JC, Maurer R, Werder K von, Torhorst J, Klijn JGM, Lamberts SWJ (1987) Somatostatin receptors in human endocrine tumors. Cancer Res 47:551-558

32. Senter PD, Saulnier MG, Schreiber GJ, Hirschberg DL, Brown JB, Hellström I, Hellström KE (1988) Anti-tumor effects of antibody-alkaline phosphatase conjugates in combination with etoposide phosphate. Proc Natl Acad Sci USA 85:4842-4846

33. Shulman M, Wilde CD, Köhler G (1978) A better cell for making hybridomas secreting specific antibodies. Nature 276:269-271

34. Schwarz A, Steinstraesser A (1987) A novel approach to Tc-99m labelled monoclonal antibodies. J Nucl Med 28:721

35. Stanley CJ, Paris F, Plumb A, Webb A, Johannson A (1985) Enzyme amplification: a new technique for enhancing the speed and sensitivity of enzyme immunoassays. Int Commission on Radiation Protection 3:44-47

36. Steinstraesser A, Seidel L, Schwarz A, Kuhlmann L, Bosslet K (1988) Immunszintigraphie mit monoklonalen Antikörpern. Diagnose und Labor 38:49-60

37. Thomas GD, Chappell MJ, Dykes PW, Ramfden PB, Godfrey KR, Ellis JRM, Bradwell AR (1989) Effect of dose, molecular size, affinity and protein binding on tumour uptake of antibody or ligand. Biomathematical model. Cancer Res 49:3290-3296

38. Vecchio S del, Reynolds JC, Carrasqiullo JA, Blasberg RG, Neumann RD, Lotze MT, Bryant GJ, Farkas RJ, Larson SM (1989) Local distribution and concentration of intravenously injected ^{131}I-9.2.27 monoclonal antibody in human malignant melanoma. Cancer Res 49:2783-2789

39. Ward ES, Güssow D, Griffiths AD, Jones PT, Winter G (1989) Binding activities of a repertoire of single immunoglobulin variable domains secreted from Escherichia coli. Nature 341:544-546

ANTIMYOSIN ANTIBODY IMAGING IN MYOCARDIAL INFARCTION

S. Bhattacharya and A. Lahiri

Introduction

Antimyosin (Myoscint TM Centocor Inc. Malvern PA) is a Fab fragment of a specific antibody to myosin heavy chains that binds to necrotic cardiac myocytes. Planar or single photon emission computed tomography (SPECT) techniques using Indium-111 labelled antibody have been used for the clinical detection of myocardial necrosis, both in acute myocardial infarction, and in myocarditis. This article reviews the role of antimyosin (AM) imaging in myocardial infarction diagnosis and risk stratification.

Antimyosin Imaging in the Diagnosis of Acute Myocardial Infarction

The specificity and sensitivity of antimyosin binding to necrotic myocardium has been documented convincingly at multiple levels: studies in cultured myocytes, in vivo animal studies, and finally in clinical studies of patients presenting with acute myocardial ischaemia.

Specificity and Sensitivity

Studies at the Cellular Level. Khaw and co-workers (1-5) demonstrated in cultured myocytes that antimyosin uptake is specific for myocyte necrosis. Scanning EM studies with antimyosin labelled polystyrene spheres (1-Angstrom unit diameter) demonstrate binding to defects in the cell membrane, where cellular contents are exposed; cells showing such binding are not viable, and fail to grow in cell culture; and antimyosin localisation is in myocytes identified as necrotic by haematoxylin and eosin staining.

In Vivo Studies. Animal experiments have shown that there is good correlation between the infarcted areas delineated by antimyosin, 99mTc-pyrophosphate, thallium 201, and by triphenyl tetrazolium chloride (TTC) (6,7) although pyrophosphate persistently overestimates the infarct size by being taken up into areas of viable but compromised myocardium. Using a dual isotope imaging technique, Narula et al (8) have recently demonstrated that intra-coronary

R. P. Baum et al. (eds.), Clinical Use of Antibodies, 69–83.

administration of the membrane stabilising agent trifluoperazine (TEP) simultaneously with reperfusion produces a reduction in the infarct size as measured by antimyosin imaging. This suggests that ischaemic myocardium while binding antimyosin may still remain potentially viable and offers an explanation for the positive scans seen in patients with unstable angina (see below). However according to experiments done by Nedelman et al (9), no antimyosin uptake could be demonstrated in severely ischemic stunned myocardium produced by a 15-minute occlusion of the left anterior descending coronary artery. Further studies need to be performed to resolve this controversy.

Autoradiography and Histopathologic Correlations in Humans. At Northwick Park we have studied two patients injected with antimyosin who died soon afterwards (due to cardia rupture at the site of myocardial necrosis) enabling a direct auto-radiographic and histopathologic correlation (10-11). Autoradiography was performed on bread-slice sections of the heart, which were subsequently stained with TTC to delineate the histopathological extent of myocardial necrosis. Excellent correlations obtained with the two different methods (Figure 1) confirm the accuracy of antimyosin uptake in demarcating infarcted myocardium. These studies also showed that antimyosin uptake occurred at histopathologically documented necrotic sites remote from the infarct related artery.

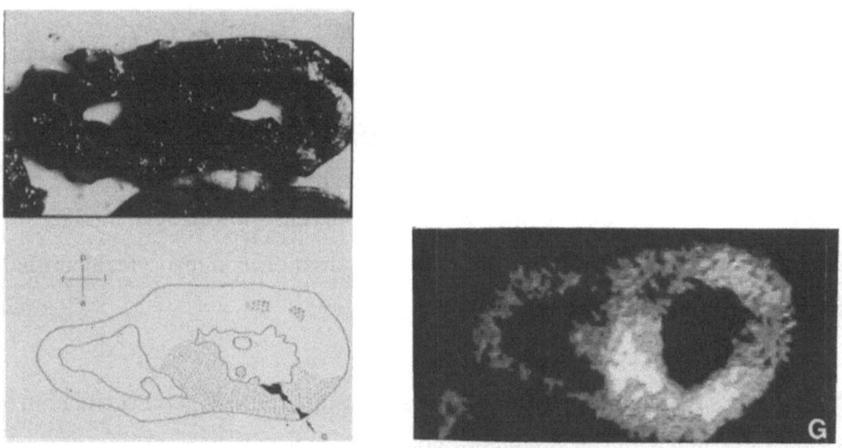

Fig.1 Bread-slice section of the heart in a patient with anterior wall MI injected with In-111 antimyosin prior to death. Top: the macroscopic appearance of antero-septal MI is clearly visualised. Middle: Diagrammatic representation of TTC/histopathology showing anterior necrosis and small islands of remote necrosis in the posterior wall. Bottom: autoradiographyof

the same slice showing close correlation between antimyosin and histopathology.

Clinical Studies. A number of large clinical studies (Table 1) have now confirmed the high sensitivity and specificity of antimyosin imaging for the diagnosis of myocardial infarction. Antimyosin uptake in patients with unstable angina suggest that either focal myocardial necrosis has occurred that was missed by EGG and serial cardiac enzymes or that antimyosin uptake can occur in ischaemic myocardium without necrosis. Experiments in animals are currently under way to explore this last possibility, and their conflicting preliminary results have been referred to earlier. The two false positive results in the multicentre study occurred in patients who had previous infarctions, and probably represented delayed positive images (see following section).

Table 1 Summary of clinical studies

Diagnosis	Pos	Neg	Sensitivity
Antimyosin Study Group (9)			
Q Wave MI	190	12	
Non-Q MI	45	10	
All MIs	235	22	91.4%
Unstable Angina	20	21	
Non-ischaemic	2	40	

Specificity for MI or unstable angina = 1- (2/42 = 95.2%
Predictive value of a positive scan for MI given a history of chest pain >30 mins considered to be due to myocardial ischaemia = 235/257 = 0.91.
Predictive value of a negative scan for non-MI chest pain = 61/83 = 0.74

Diagnosis	Pos	Neg	Sensitivity
Volpini et al 1989 (10)			
Acute MI	49	1	98%
Non MI chest pain	1	6	
Healthy volunteers	0	10	
Johnson et al 19989 (11)			
Acute MI	46	4	92%
Khaw et al 1987 (12)			
Acute MI	52	2	96.3%

Positive

Pos: positive scans; **Neg**: Negative scans

Clinical Scanning Techniques

At Northwick Park Hospital, antimyosin (2mCi of In-111 labelled antimyosin Fab) is injected intravenously after testing for radiochemical purity using instant thin layer chromatography. Planar imaging is performed routinely in three views (anterior, 45° LAO and 70° LAO or left lateral) using a gamma scintillation camera (IGE 400AT, Radlett UK) at 24 and at 48 hours post injection, data being acquired in digital format. Each image is acquired for 10 minutes, positioning the heart fully in the field of view, and minimizing the amount of liver uptake. Dual photopeaks of 173 and 247 Kev are used with symmetric 20% windows . For SPECT imaging, 64 frames are acquired over 180° from RAO to LPO positions, at 30 seconds per frame. The total time required is approximately 30 minutes. Diagnostic quality images are obtained at 24 to 48 hours post injection due to the presence of cardiac blood pool in scans performed earlier.

The difficulty in quantifying the extent of antimyosin uptake on planar images by computer edge definition methods has led to the development of a semi-quantitative technique which is based on the bull's eye technique commonly used in thallium-201 imaging (Figures 2 and 3) The extent of antimyosin uptake in each of three views is related to a single polar coordinate map or bull's eye, composed of 18 segments. The uptake of antimyosin can then be related to one of the major coronary vascular beds.

Delayed Positive Images and Heart Lung Ratio

Persistent uptake of antimyosin in infarcted areas has been observed when imaging is performed from 4 to 270 days post infarction (Figure 4) (12,13).

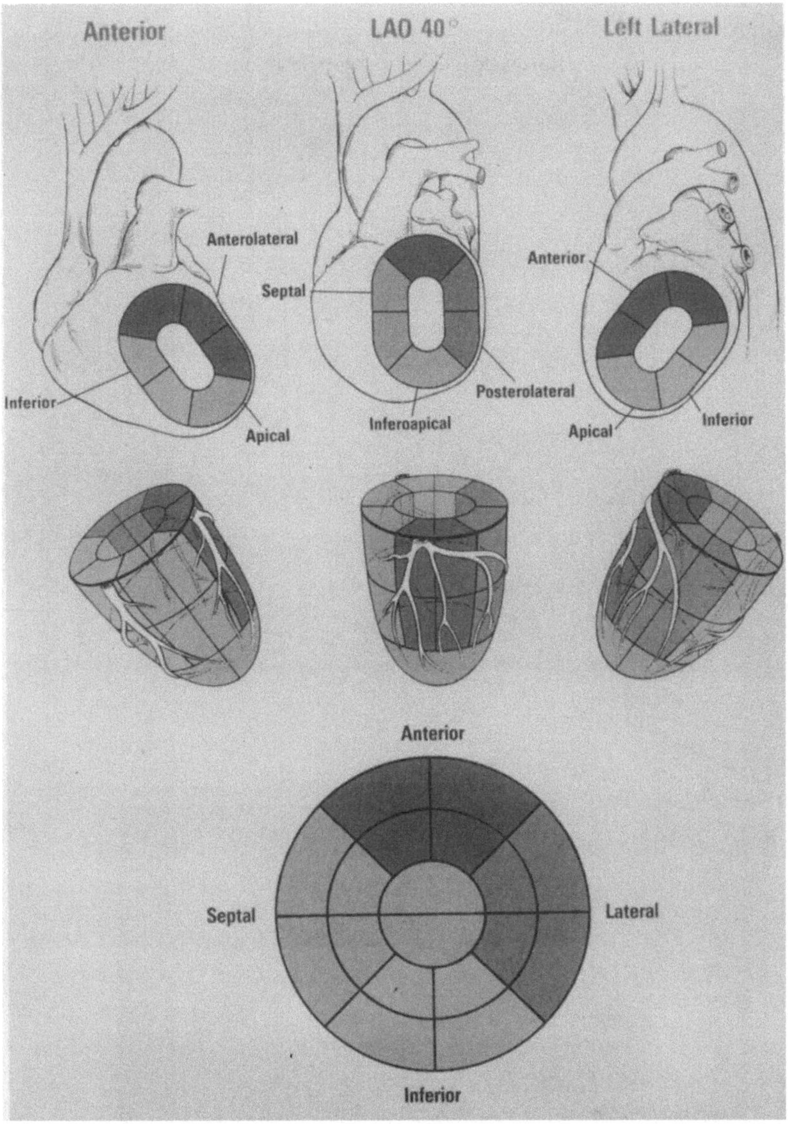

Fig.2 Bullseye technique: construction of a bullseye image from the three planar scans

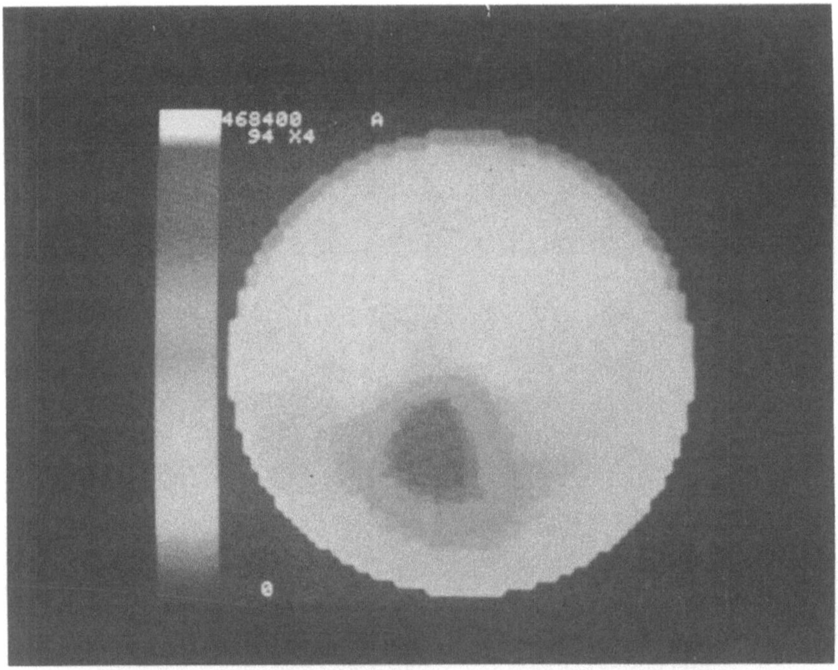

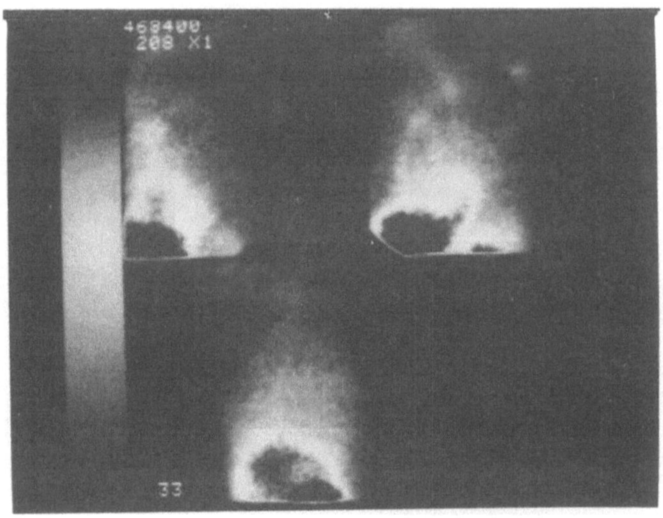

Fig. 3a and 3b Small inferior myocardial infarction clearly demonstrated by the bullseye (3a) but not well seen on the planar scans (3b).

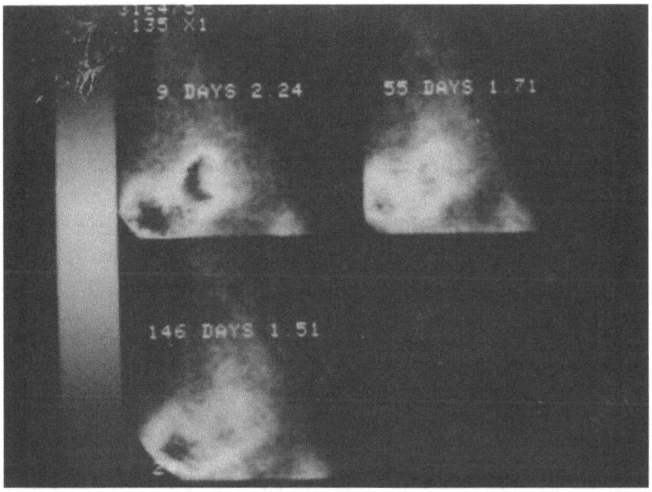

Fig.4 Delayed positive uptake. Serial LAO images with In-111 antimyosin obtained at days 9.55 and post infarction showing diminishing uptake of antimyosin and progressive reduction in the heart/lung ratio.

The mechanism for this delayed uptake is not clear, but it may be due to either persistence of myosin epitopes (myosin being an insoluble protein), ongoing necrosis in islands of ischaemic tissue in the previously infarcted zone, or non specific accumulation of antibody in inflamed and oedematous tissue, or perhaps a combination of these mechanisms. This phenomenon widens the diagnostic time window, allowing the accurate diagnosis of myocardial infarction up to 12 weeks post infarction. This would be clinically important in patients where there is a post history of undiagnosed chest pain and no diagnostic EGG changes at the time of examination. Such patients frequently present to the cardiologist at the time of a pre-anaesthetic evaluation, and a negative scan would allow as more confident decision to proceed with their surgery.

However, persistent uptake also results in difficulty in distinguishing old from fresh myocardial necrosis. Liu et al (14) have shown that a heart/lung ratio greater than 2 (measured using a 9 x 9 pixel region of interest over the region of peak myocardial uptake, at 24 hours post antimyosin injection) suggests recent myocardial necrosis. In serial antimyosin images performed on the same patient, there is a progressive decrease in the heart/lung ratio. This quantitative method may therefore be used to distinguish recent versus old infarcts.

Diagnosis in 'Gray Zone' Individuals

Clinicians are frequently beset by the problem of patients presenting with chest pains, but with no diagnostic EGG changes, and such patients may constitute up to 10-15% of the total. Jain et al (15) recently have described 7 patients presenting with chest pains and no serial EGG change, but with raised peak CK. All 7 patients had infarction diagnosed by antimyosin imaging (Figure 5). These patients therefore represent an important group in whom antimyosin imaging can be used to estimate infarct size and prognosis.

Dual Isotope Imaging and the Detection of Myocardium at Risk

Dual isotope imaging i.e. In-111 antimyosin combined with an agent that images myocardial perfusion such as Thallium-201 or 99mTC-sestamibi is a new technique that has certain advantages. Quantitative data on the relative myocardial involvement (i.e. ratio of infarcted to total myocardium) cannot be easily obtained by planar imaging, as the normal myocardium does not take up antimyosin. SPECT images are useful in infarct localisation in cases where there is 'shine-through' on the planar image.

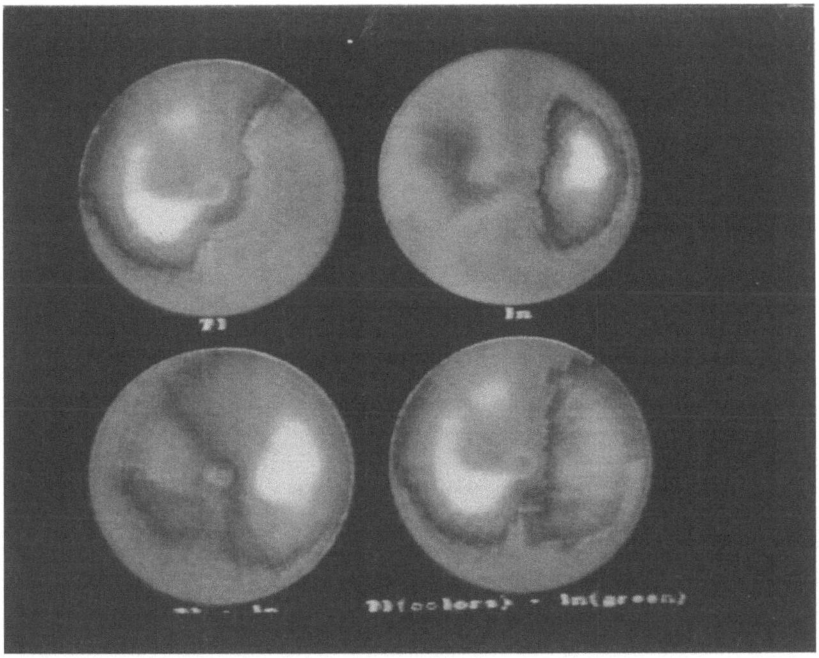

Fig.5 Dual isotope imaging with thallium-201 and Indium-111 antimyosin in a patient with a lateral wall infarction. Top left: thallium bullseye showing extensive lateral and inferior wall defect. Top tight: antimyosin uptake in the lateral wall. Bottom right: composite thallium and antimyosin image with antimyosin uptake in green. An extensive inferior perfusion defect in the absence of necrosis (mismatch) suggests the presence of 'hibernating' myocardium. At angiography the patient had a totally occluded circumflex artery and a 90% stenosis in the right coronary artery, which was dilated successfully by PTCA.

Reconstruction of SPECT images however requires cardiac anatomical references (16), which are not available with standard antimyosin images when the infarct size is small. Using a dual isotope technique, and superimposing the perfusion and the antimyosin images allows the delineation of cardia landmarks, and also allows visualisation of the non-infarcted myocardium. Based on the available experience (17-19) we have summarised the diagnostic patterns observed with this technique in patients with acute coronary syndromes (Table 2 and Figure 5).

TABLE 2 - Diagnostic patterns with dual isotope imaging

Diagnosis	In-111 AM Uptake	Perfusion Defect	Akinesia
Irreversible damage	Matching	Matching	Matching
Non-transmural MI (Overlap)	Large	Small	Variable
Reperfused myocardium (Stunned)	Small	Small	Large
Hibernating myocardium (Mismatch)	Small	Large	Large
Acute Ischaemia (Mismatch)	Small	Large	Small
Remote Infarction	Small	Nil	Small

Dual isotope imaging is valuable in distinguishing transmural from non-transmural infarction which is suggested by the presence of some perfusion agent uptake in the area of anti-myosin uptake, whereas in transmural infarction there is no perfusion at the site of necrosis. These results need confirmation by histopathologic techniques. Hibernating myocardium describes those viable myocardial areas which are poorly perfused and at risk, and consequently are likely to improve with successful revascularisation. A technique to detect it is therefore likely to be clinically important. Remote infarction (19) refers to the uptake of antimyosin in areas distinct from the main site of uptake. This pattern was described in patients with a first Q-wave infarct, thus excluding the possibility of a previous infarction being responsible. No perfusion defect was found at these remote sites, suggesting mechanisms other than total or subtotal coronary occlusion being responsible. This was further corroborated by the finding that 3 patients had only single vessel disease, with a patent artery supplying the area of remote infarction. Possible mechanisms of remote infarction are spasm of the non-infarct artery, or increased myocardial oxygen demand due to poor left ventricular function, neuroendocrine mechanisms, and altered left ventricular geometry secondary to a large infarction.

RISK STRATIFICATION AND PROGNOSIS

The persistence of radioactivity in the blood pool for up to 24 hours following antimyosin injection impedes detection of positive scans early in the course of a myocardial infarction. Consequently, antimyosin imaging, at least with currently available preparations is unlikely to be of much importance in planning thrombolytic or other acute therapies. However, the scintigraphic image offers the unique opportunity to accurately quantify infarct size and assess prognosis.

Infarct Size and Prognosis

Quantification of infarct size - Autoradiographic and histopathologic correlations in clinical studies of patients dying of M1 following antimyosin injection, have shown that both infarct size as well as location can be accurately predicted by antimyosin imaging (10,11). Clinical studies have also shown that the extent of antimyosin uptake is strongly correlated with traditional indicators of infarct size including ECG, 99mTc-pyrophosphateimaging, peak CK-MB, the size of thallium-201 perfusion defect and, is inversely correlated with injection, fraction and wall motion scores obtained from gated blood pool scans (20-22). Antimyosin imaging therefore allows direct scintigraphic assessment of infarct size and consequently is likely to be an important prognostic indicator in patients with chest pains.

PrognosticImportantof AntimyosinUptake - This was studied in a large multicentrestudy (23) of patients presenting with a suspected myocardial infarction. There was a highly significant correlation between the number of segments of antimyosin uptake and the incidence of subsequentcardia death and non-fatal myocardialinfarction. The risk of a cardiac event within the next 60-days was 26% in patients with extensive uptake (>10/18 segments), compared to about 5% in patients with in those with less than 10 or no segments showing uptake of antimyosin. Extensive antimyosin uptake has superior prognostic value compared with other predictors of cardiac risk which included Killip class, age, Q wave myocardial infarction, recurrentischaemia and peak CK. The sensitivityand specificityof extensiveantimyosin uptake in identifying high risk patients was 43% and 89% respectively

Prognostic Important of Perfusion and Necrosis Mismatch and Overlap. The finding of a significant mismatch between the perfusion and the antimyosin images i.e. the presence of perfusion defects in the absence of antimyosin uptake is predictive for recurrent ischaemia. Thus, of 24 patients with acute M1 studied by Johnson et al (18), 7 who had no evidence of mismatch did not develop any further ischaemic events (defined as in-hospital infarct extension, recurrent angina or ischaemia on pre-dischargestress test or 6 months thallium stress test).Of the remaining 17 patients, 13 had mismatching thallium defects, and 4 had thallium-antimyosin overlap i.e. areas with anti-myosin uptake that have smaller or no corresponding perfusion defect. 14 of these 17 patients went on to have further episodes of ischaemia, and multivessel disease was found in 12 of 13 patients who underwent angiography.

SimultaneousAssessmentof Left VentricularFunction.

Recent studies (24) have shown that it is possible to use the early blood pool phase following an antimyosin injection to determine left ventricular ejection fraction and recognise regional wall motion abnormalities by performing equilibrium radionuclide ventriculography. The regional wall motion abnormalities and the injection fraction correlate closely ($r=0.95, p<0.001$) with the antimyosin uptake, and this method may improve prognostic risk stratification using a single radionuclide injection.

CONCLUSIONS

Antimyosin imaging will undoubtedly have a major role in the risk stratificationof patients who have had a recent acute coronary episode, especially with the advent of dual isotope imaging techniques which allows the rapid detection of myocardium at risk. Patients in the 'gray zone' are also likely to benefit from this technique as it allows a method of diagnosis and infarct sizing. It is obviously important to be able to obtain diagnostic quality images as soon as possible using antimyosin, and two recent advances deserve mention. 99mTc-labelled antimyosin, which has a more rapid clearance from the blood pool, and superior imaging qualities compared to Indium-111 (not to mention being cheaper) has recently entered the clinical trial phase, and the results appear promising. More specific diagnostic images may also be obtained with the polylysinated antibody recently developed by Khaw and colleagues (15) which has a higher specificity for myosin owing to its net negative charge.

It is also important to develop agents that can image active coronary lesions and developing thrombi: trials with such agents which include labelled tissue plasminogen activator (26), antifibrin antibodies, and antibodies to the GMP140 protein (S12) (27) which is a marker for activated platelets and endothelial cells are already in progress. With the availability of potent thrombolytic and anti-platelet therapy (e.g 7E3 and RGDY) it is likely that our efforts as clinical cardiologists will be directed at the early diagnosis and therapy of coronary thrombosis before the development of irreversible myocardial necrosis.

References

1. Khaw B.A.et al(1979) Specificity of localisation of myosin-specific antibody fragments in experimental myocardial infarction: histologic, histochemical, autoradiographic and scintigraphic studies. Circulation 60, 1527-1531

2. Frame L.H et al (1983) Early membrane damage during coronary reperfusion in dogs: detection by radiolabelled anticardiac myosin (Fab')^2 J.Clin.Invest/ 72, 535-544

3. khaw B.A.et al (1980) Myocardial infarct imaging of antibodies to canine myosin with Indium-111-diethylene-triaminepentaacetic acid, Science 209, 295-297

4. Khaw B.A. et al (1984) Monoclonal antibody to cardiac myosin: imaging of experimental myocardial infarction, Hybridoma 3,11-23

5. Khaw B.A et al (1982) Myocardial injury: quantification by cell sorting initiated with antimyosin fluorescent spheres, Science 217: 1050-1053

6. Khaw B.A. et al (1987) Myocardial damage delineated by indium-111 antimyosin Fab and technetium-99m pyrophosphate. J.Nucl.Med.28: 76-82

7. Johnson L.L. et al (1987) Measurementof infarct size and percentagemyocardium infarcted in a dog preparation with single photon-emission computed tomography, thallium-201 and indium 111-monoclonal antimyosin Fab. Circulation 76: 181-190

8. Narula J et al (1990) Documentation of re perfusion myocardial injury by dual radio-labelled anti-myosin imaging: reversibility by membrane stabilising agent.J.Nucl.Med.31:805 (Abstract)

9. Nedelman M.A et al (1990) Evaluation of antimyosin uptake in reversibly injured ('stunned) myocardium J.Nucl.Med.31: 783 (Abstract)

10. Jain D. et al (1988) Postmortem correlation between histopathologic and autoradiographic extent of myocardial necrosis detected by 111-In-antimyosinimaging in a patients with acute myocardial infarction.Am.J.CardiacImaging 2: 158-161

11. Jain D et al (1990) Indium-111 antimyosin images compared with triphenyl tetrazolium chloride staining in a patient six days after myocardial infarction.J.Nucl.Med.31:231-233

12. Tamaki N et al (1989)(Clinical trial of 111-In-antimyosinantibody imaging (3) Comparison with 99mTc-pyrophosphateimaging) Kaku Igaku 26: 1199-1205

13. Jain D et al (1989) Late imaging of myocardial infarction with In-111 antimyosin antibodies. Eur.J.Nucl.Med. 15: 474 (Abstract)

14. Liu X.J et al (1990) A quantitative method for assessing age of myocardial infarction from antimyosin images.J.Nucl.Med. 31: 782 (Abstract)

15. Jain D et al (1990) Immunoscintigraphyfor the detection of acute myocardial infarction in the absence of electrocardiographicchanges.Br.Med.J.300:151-153

16. Morguet A et al (1989) Tc-99m methoxy-isobutyl-isonitrile (MIBI) for anatomical landmarking in imaging acute myocardial infarction (AMI) with antimyosin Fab (AM Fab) J.Nucl.Med.30: 800 (Abstract)

17. Knapp W.H. et al (1989) In-111 antimyosin antibodies and Tc-99m-MIBI for assessment of post-infarction myocardial viability.J.Nucl.Med. 30: 800 (Abstract)

18. Johnson L.L. and Seldin D.W. (1989) The role of antimyosin antibodies in acute myocardial infarction. Semin.Nucl.Med. 19: 238-246

19. Jain D et al (1988) Discordance between In-111 antimyosin uptake, regional perfusion and wall motion abnormalities in acute Q-wave myocardial infarction. Circulation 78: Supply.11 431 (Abstract)

20. Khaw B.A. et al (1989) Scintigraphic quantification of myocardial necrosis in patients after intravenous injection of myosin-specific antibody. Circulation 74: 501-508

21. Antunes M.L. et al (1989) Measurement of acute Q-wave myocardial infarct size with single photon emission computed tomography imaging of indium-111 antimyosin. Am.J.Cardiol.63: 777-783

22. Volpini M. et al (1989) Diagnosis of acute myocardial infarction by indium-111 antimyosin antibodies and correlation with the traditional techniques for the evaluation of extent and localisation. Am J.Cardiol.63: 7-13

23. Berger H. et al (1988) Antimyosin imaging in patients with ischemic chest pain: initial results of phase 111 multicentre trial.J.Nucl.Med.29 805 (Abstract)

24. Lahiri A. et al (1990) Combined assessment of myocardial necrosis and left ventricular function with a single dose of In-111 antimyosin J.Nucl.Med. 31: 841 (Abstract)

25. Khaw B.A. et al (1989) Modification of monoclonal antimyosin antibody: enhanced specificity of localisation and scintigraphic visualisation in acute experimental myocardial infarction. J.Mol.Cell Cardiol. 21: Supply 1. 31-35

26. Kader K.L. et al (1990) Rapid localaisation of In-111 labelled recombinant tissue plasminogen activator in a rabbit thrombosis model J.Nucl.Med.31: 805 (Abstract)

27. Chouraqui P. et al (1990) Successful in vivo visualisation of occlusive arterial thrombi by Tc-99m labelled monoclonal antibody against activated platelets. J.Nucl.Med. 30: 713 (Abstract)

ANTIMYOSIN BASED RADIOIMMUNODETECTION OF MYOCARDITIS CARDIOMYOPATHY AND CARDIAC TRANSPLANT REJECTION

I.Carrio

111-Indium-Antimyosin specifically binds to exposed cardiac myosin and is used to precisely delineate myocardial necrosis in patients with myocardial infarct. Antimyosin is also an appropriate method to assess the presence of myocyte damage in cardiomyopathy and after heart transplantation, as cell necrosis can be present in variable degrees in both situations.

The calculation of a heart to lung ratio (HLR) dividing average counts per pixel in the myocardium by average counts per pixel in the lungs (1) is useful to express the degree of antimyosin uptake. Changes in the degree of antimyosin uptake can document either improvement or worsening of the disease, or can be used to assess the response to immunosuppressive treatment.

Myocarditis

The gold standard to diagnose myocarditis remains right ventricular endomyocardial biopsy, a method which can lack sensitivity due to sampling error. Diagnosis of active myocarditis is still made by clinical symptoms, and decisions regarding therapy are often taken without a positive biopsy. There is, therefore, a need for a noninvasive method to assess the extent of myocardial damage in these patients.

In patients with suspicion of acute myocarditis, positive antimyosin scans show diffuse antimyosin uptake in the myocardium. In 13 patients with suspected acute myocarditis (heart failure of less than 6 months or acute onset), antimyosin studies were positive in 11 (Carrio). HRL was 2.0±0.5; indicating the presence of active cell damage in this group despite the small proportion of positive right ventricular endomyocardial biopsy (4 of 13). In the study by Yasuda et al.(2) 17 of 28 patients with suspected acute myocarditis had positive antimyosin scans, and 9 of 28 had positive biopsies. These results indicate a superior sensitivity of antimyosin scans compared to right ventricular endomyocardial biopsy in the detection of myocardial damage in these patients. Antimyosin scans are a reliable method for the evaluation of patients suspected of having myocarditis. A positive scan may indicate the need for

R. P. Baum et al. (eds.), Clinical Use of Antibodies, 85–89.

endomyocardial biopsy, while patients who present with a negative scan can avoid biopsy.

Chronic Idiopathic Dilated Cardiomyopathy

The clinical course of dilated cardiomyopathy is exceedingly variable. A few patients present an illness that resolves spontaneously or with immunosuppressive treatment; in others the illness evolves rapidly, within months, and the patient eventually dies or requires transplantation. Most patients follow a long-term clinical course. The natural history of dilated cardiomyopathy is that of a steady deterioration of functional class; the survival curves indicate a downhill course, especially during the first years after the diagnosis is made.

The progressive nature of dilated cardiomyopathy has been explained as being a result of the long-term exhaustion of compensatory mechanisms initiated by a decrease in myocardial cell mass. However, necropsy studies in patients with this condition seldom reveal myocardial necrosis; in fact, there is a striking lack of correlation between the microscopic findings and the degree of cardiac disfunction in patients with end-stage dilated cardiomyopathy.

In a study to assess the presence of antimyosin uptake in patients with chronic idiopathic dilated cardiomyopathy(3), three groups were studied: 17 patients with chronic (>12 months) idiopathic dilated cardiomyopathy, 12 patients with a large, poorly contracting left ventricle not due to dilated cardiomyopathy (control patients) and 8 normal individuals. The patients in the cardiomyopathy and control groups showed a similar degree of clinical functional impairment. The mean HLR in the cardiomyopathy group was 1.83±0.36 (range 1.40 to 2.80), a value significantly higher than that obtained in the control patients without cardiomyopathy (mean 1.46±0.13, range 1.31 to 1.60) or normal subjects (mean 1.46±0.04, range 1.38 to 1.5) ($p<0.01$). No difference in the HLR was noted between the normal subjects and control patients. Abnormal antimyosin uptake was seen in 12 (70%) of the 17 patients with cardiomyopathy.

These results indicate 1) that there is a high prevalence of antimyosin uptake in patients with stable chronic idiopathic dilated cardiomyopathy, and 2) that positive antimyosin studies are not due to left ventricular dilation or to the consequences of heart failure, as a similar cardiac impairment was present in the control groups of patients with left ventricular dilation and dysfunction.

Myocardial uptake of antimyosin in chronic dilated cardiomyopathy reflects the presence of on going myocyte damage in these patients. Antimyosin scans identify patients who have antimyosin uptake and those who have a negative scan. Continual myocardial uptake could explain the steady clinical deterioration in some patients with dilated cardiomyopathy, and the stable course in others without such myocardial uptake. It is possible that patients with dilated cardiomyopathy and a positive antimyosin study might respond to some form of therapy (i.e. immunosuppression) directed to halt the process, whereas those with absent uptake would not.

Doxorubicin Cardiotoxicity

Patients under doxorubicin therapy need close cardiac monitoring to identify those at risk of developing heart failure when the schedule of doses can still be modified. Patients at risk can receive high cumulative doses if the schedule of administration is modified to avoid heart failure. The histologic changes related to doxorubicin toxicity consist in the presence of degenerative myocytes and interstitial fibrosis.

To assess if antimyosin scans were able to detect myocardial damage after chemotherapy including doxorubicin, antimyosin scans were performed after 10 cycles of doxorubicin with a total cumulative dose of 500 mg/m^2 (treatment also included cyclophosphamide and 5-fluorouracil) in 20 women with advanced breast cancer (4). Left ventricular ejection fraction was determined before and after treatment. The ejection fraction decreased 5% after chemotherapy in 8 of 20 (40%) patients. Seventeen of 20 (85%) patients presented with antimyosin uptake in the myocardium ($p<0.01$). Patients with decrease in ejection fraction presented with more intense antimyosin uptake (HLR of 2.11±0.10 versus 1.70−±0.16 ($p<0.01$). Nine of 12 patients without decrease in ejection fraction presented with antimyosin uptake. HLR values correlated with ejection fraction values after chemotherapy ($r=-0.47$, $p<0.05$).

	EF before	EF after	HRL
n=12	57.7±7.3	58.2±7.5	1.70±0.16
n= 8	59.3±6.3	46.7±9.2 *	2.11±0.10 *

*: $p<0.01$

Myocardial antimyosin uptake after chemotherapy including doxorubicin indicates the presence of myocardial damage in these patients, although only in a small proportion to the extent necessary to deteriorate function. Antimyosin scans may be a sensitive method to monitor cardiotoxicity in patients under doxorubicin therapy.

Heart Transplantation

Diagnosis of cardiac allograft rejection after heart transplantationis based on interpretation of endomyocardial biopsy. Repeat biopsies are required during the first year. This is inconvenient and the cost is high. Antimyosin scans provide a noninvasive method to detect cardiac rejection and to assess the time course of myocyte damage after transplantation(5,6,7).

Antimyosin uptake after transplantationwas correlatedwith results of endomyocardialbiopsy in 62 patients, 7 days to 40 months after transplantation. In 18 patients with endomyocardial biopsy indicating rejection (inflammatory cell infiltration and myocyte necrosis), HLR was 1.90±0.34. In 23 patients with biopsy showing inflammatory infiltrates but without myocyte damage , HLR was 1.77±0.25. In 21 patients with normal biopsy, HLR was 1.61±0.20 ($p=0.001$)

Patients with repeat studies after transplantation presented with initially high HLR which tended to decrease with time (studies performed 1-3 months after transplantation, HLR of 1.89±0.3; studies performed > 12 months HLR of 1.65±2, $p<0.01$), showing that after transplantation lesional myocardial activity tends to decrease gradually. Persistence of high HLR values correlated with persistent rejection activity detected at biopsy and implied a poor prognosis. Patients who normalised their HLR during follow-up composed a low risk group.

Eight of 12 patients with HLR>1.58 one year after transplantation, presented with biopsy proven rejection (17 episodes) during subsequent follow-up. One of 9 patients with HLR 1.58 one year after transplantation, presented with 1 episode of biopsy proven rejection during subsequent follow-up ($p=0.01$). The number of rejection episodes per patient during follow-up correlated with HLR one year after transplantation($r=0.64$; $p<0.01$). The 9 patients with HLR 1.58 had 0.1 episodes of rejection per patient (1 episode). Seven patients with HLR>1.58 1.75 had 1.28 episodes of rejection per patient (9 episodes). Five patients with HLR>1.75 had 1.6 episodes of rejection per patient during follow-up (8 episodes) ($p<0.05$)

Patterns of antimyosin uptake are useful in defining clinical outcome and determining patient management. Early after transplantation, persistence or increase in myocardial antimyosin uptake indicates rejection-relatedcomplications. When high HLR persist after one year, despite an apparently good clinical course, careful screening for abnormal rejection is required. Patients who normalise HLR during follow-up are in a low risk group; in these circumstances noninvasive follow-up with antimyosin studies might be justified.

References

1. Carrio I. et al.[1988] Indium-111 antimyosin scintigraphy to assess myocardial damage in patients with suspected myocarditis and cardiac rejection.J.Nucl.Med.1892-1990

2. Yasuda T. et al.[1987] Indium-111 monoclonal antimyosin antibody imaging in the diagnosis of acute myocarditis. Circulation.76: 306-311

3. Obrador D. et al.[1989] High prevalence of myocardial monoclonal antimyosin antibody uptake in patients with chronic idiopathic dilated cardiomyopathy. J.Am.Coll.Cardiol. 13: 1289-1293

4. Estorch M. et al.[1989] 111-In-Antimyosin myocardial uptake in patients under adriamycin therapy for advanced breast cancer. Eur.J.Nucl.Med.8.465

5. Ballester M et al.[1988] Patterns of evolution of myocyte damage after human heart transplantation detected by Indium-111 monoclonal antimyosin.Am.J.Cardiol.62:623-627

6. Baum R.P. et al.[1989] In-111 Antimyosin Fab monoclonal antibody imaging in the diagnosis of acute transplant rejection. J.Nucl.Med.5.847

7. Carrio I. et al.[1989] Noninvasive follow-up of heart transplant patients with quantitative In-111-Antimyosin scintigraphy. J.Nucl.Med.5.862.

RECENT ADVANCES IN THE USE OF RADIOLABELLED MONOCLONAL ANTIBODIES IN THE MANAGEMENT OF OVARIAN CANCER.

M.Granowska, K.E.Britton, S.J.Mather, M.Naeem, T.Jobling, J.H.Shepherd

Introduction

Ovarian Cancer is a debilitating disease. It usually presents in an advanced state and then requires radical surgery and repeated courses of chemotherapy. It is the second most common cause of death due to cancer in women.

The advances in the management of ovarian cancer through the use of radiolabelled antibodies, radioimmunoscintigraphy,RIS, are several. They include the better evaluation of the responses to chemotherapy before second look surgery, in particular the demonstration of whether a mass seen radiologically has viable tumour or not (1) and the detection of recurrences not visible on X-ray CT or ultrasound (2). This is leading to a reduction in the application of second look surgery to determine the need for further chemotherapy. There is the demonstration of the sites of tumour when a rise in a serum marker is detected (3) and indeed tumour detection without such a rise in serum markers is increasingly noted using RIS (4). The evaluation of ultrasound screened pelvic lesions in women by RIS is needed to seek to reduce the number of unnecessary operations on well women in whom a pelvic lesion is found. In a recent study ultrasound led to operations in 324 women out of 5000 screened of whom only nine had ovarian cancer (5).

These practical and potential clinical advances are coming about through considerable technical advances. There has been an evolution in the radiolabel for RIS from I-131 through I-123 (6) and In-111 (7) to Tc-99m (8,9) and this has been done in part to an improvement in labelling techniques. The stability of the In-111 label on the antibody has been increased from the use of the cyclic anhydride of DTPA (10) to the use of 'backbone' substitutes such as benzyl DTPA (11), to the use of macrocycles with a 12 membered ring (12). This improvement in the stability of the In-111 antibody combination has not, unfortunately, led to significant reduction in liver uptake. The move from the pre-tinning of antibody for Tc-99m labelling (13) to the Schwarz technique (14) and its modifications (15) has given a Tc-99m labelled antibody that is stable in vivo without the need for thyroid blockade. For therapy the

R. P. Baum et al. (eds.), Clinical Use of Antibodies, 91–110.

advance has been from I-131 to Y-90 (16) and hopefully to P32 (17).

The monoclonal antibodies used for RIS have also evolved from HMFG 1 & 2 (against the human milk fat globule glycoprotein antigen of the epithelial surface lining of the lactiferous ducts of the breast but present in the ovarian and gastrointestinal epithelia (18)) to SM3 against the deglycosylated 'stripped' mucin core protein (19) with the intention of reducing its reactivity with benign tumours. OVTL3 is a new antibody for ovarian cancer RIS with good specifity for malignant ovarian tumours (20).

The development of SM3 was based on the postulate that there is aberrant glycosylation of mucin glycoproteins in malignant tissue in contrast to benign or normal tissue with fully processed mucin characteristic of normal differentiation. Therefore the HMFG antigen was purified by affinity chromatographyand the mucin glycoproteinwas stripped of its carbohydrate using hydrogen fluoride. The resulting mucin core protein was used as an immunogen for the generation of a new set of monoclonal antibodies. One of these, SM3, stripped mucin antibody 3, was shown by immunoperoxidase staining to have low affinity for benign and high affinity for malignant breast tissue (19).

It was further shown that SM3 reacts with an epitope of the mucin glycoprotein containing the amino acid sequence Pro. Asp. Thr. Arg. Pro. whereas HMFG2 reacts with only the shorter sequence Asp. Thr. Arg.. The longer amino acid sequence is thought to be less exposed in the benign tissue because of the greater degree of branching and overlap of the glycosyl radicles whereas in malignant tissue, the shorter less dense glycosyl radicles enable access of the antibody to the longer sequence (21) hence the greater specificity of SM3 for malignant than benign tumours. SM3 was therefore selected for clinical trials for radioimmunoscintigraphyin breast and ovarian cancer (22).

There has been considerable improvement in image analysis from the crude subtraction of distributions of radionuclides with different energies, Tc-99m albumin from I-131 monoclonal antibodies (23) with its inherent disadvantages (24), to subtraction of the early image from the latter one (25), to kinetic analysis with probability mapping (26).

Materials and Methods

The HMG1, HMFG2 and SM3 monoclonal Antibodies were prepared in the ICRF laboratories so as to meet recommended quality assurance standards (27). The preparation was radiolabelled either with I-123, with In-111 or with Tc-99m in a purpose designed radiopharmacy under aseptic conditions.

Labelling with I-123 was with the iodogen technique (2). The iodogen is dissolved in dichloromethane to male iodogen solution and evaporated to dryness at 37^0C in sterile propylene tubes. Iodogen reagent is then coating the inside of the tube and these tubes can be stored at 5^0C for 6 months without loss of reactivity.

Once the iodogen tubes are prepared, the following technique is used for labelling. Pure ^{123}I, the mouse monoclonal antibody, SM3, 1-2 mg/ml in 10^{-5}M , Tris buffer, pH 7.4 and potassium iodide, 4 x 10^{-4}M in water are mixed in the iodogen tube. Potassium iodide is added because it is necessary to increase the ionic strength of the iodine for the labelling reaction to proceed in completion.

The mixture is left at room temperature for 10 min with gentle shaking. The mixture is decanted on to a Sephadex G-50 filtration column in a 20-ml syringe pre-washed with 1% human serum albumen in phosphate-bufferedsaline. After a 5ml void volume, the eluate is collected in 2ml aliquots, activity assayed and passed through a 0.22 micron micropore filter into sterile vials.

Quality control is undertaken using 10 ul samples from before and after gel filtration. They are spotted at an origin of 10 cm absorbent strips. These are developed in an ascending manner with 85% methanol and the radioactivity of the strips is determined. The labelling efficiency is typically over 70%. Iodinated protein is precipitated at origin and free I-123 is at solvent front. Reactivity of iodinated antibody with breast cancer cells is tested using enzyme-linked immunoabsorbentassay (ELISA). It is shown that this iodogen method leaves the active centre of the antibody intact with its avidity unaltered. This is also confirmed by a direct radioimmunoassay.

Labelling with In-111 was by the bifunctional chelate technique using the cyclic anhydride of diethylene triamine pentaacetic acid, ADTPA (10). Metal free vessels and reagents are essential. The antibody is derivatised using ADTPA using an anhydride antibody molar ratio of between two and four to one. The unbound ADTPA is separated from the protein bound DTPA by chromatography using a Superose-12 FPLC gel filtration column. The derivatised antibody is collected and aliquoted into 1mg doses and frozen for future use. Sterility and apyrogenicity tests are undertaken.

Radiolabelling is performed as follows. The vial of In-111 chloride is buffered with 5 Molar acetate solution to pH 5.5 so that the concentration of acetate is 0.5 Molar. The antibody is thawed and added drop by drop to the buffered IN-111 and the mixture is allowed to react for 20 minutes. Column chromatographyis used to separate the free Indium salts and the purity of the labelled antibody is tested using thin layer chromatography. Immunoreactivity was confirmed by ELISA testing to be over 90%. The same approach is used for labelling the monoclonal antibody with Y-90 for therapy (28).

Labelling with Tc-99m was by the Schwarz method as modified in this department (15). The S-S bonds holding the heavy chains together in the hinge region of the gamma globulin are opened using 2-mercapto ethanol, 2-ME. The antibody is concentrated by ultrafiltration to approximately 10 mg/ml. To stirred solution of antibody, sufficient 2-mercaptoethanol is added to provide a molar ratio of 1000:1, 2-ME:antibody. The mixture is incubated at room temperature for 30 minutes with continuous rotation. The reduced antibody is purified by gel filtration on Sephadex - G50 using Phosphate buffered saline as mobile phase. The antibody fractions are collated and divided into 0.5mg aliquots. These are frozen immediately at -20 deg C and stored ready for use.

When imaging is required the antibody aliquot is thawed and reconstituted using an Amerscan methylene diphosphonate, MDP, kit with 5ml 0.9% sterile saline. 50 microlitres of MDP solution are added to antibody aliquot and mixed well. Then the required amount of Tc-99m pertechnetate(700MBq approx) is added to antibody/MDP mixture, which is gently shaken for 10 minutes. The labelling efficiency is assessed by thin layer chromatography (ITLC) developed in o.9% saline and should be over 95%. If below this, the labelled antibody can be further purified by gel filtration on Sephadex G50 prior to injection. The labelled antibody is stable for some hours in vitro after preparation. This Tc-99m labelled antibody is stable in vivo. There is no thyroid uptake of Tc-99m even after 24 hours in patients who have received no thyroid blocking medication. This technique has been successfully used for four different antibodies in clinical use in this Department to date.

I-131 labelling of monoclonal antibody for therapy was undertaken using the method of Mather and Ward (29) which was developed in house. The iodogen approach requires a final column purification step which exposes the operator to an increased radiation hazard. This step is avoided with the use of N-bromo succinamide which achieves a 95% labelling efficiency without further purification.

Radioimmunoscintigraphy

Patients with suspected or known ovarian cancer who were between 30 and 75 years of age were selected for radioimmunoscintigraphyby the gynaecologicaloncologysurgeons. The studies were approved by the City and Hackney District Health Authority Ethical Committee and licenced by the Administration of Radioactive Substances Advisory Committee of the Department of Health and Social Services. The procedure was explained to each patient and signed informed consent was obtained. For those receiving I-123 SM3, potassium iodide 60mg twice daily was given orally in the day before and for three days during and after the study, which was completed within 24 hours. No special preparation was given for the patient receiving In-111 SM3 or Tc-99m SM3. No skin testing was performed so as to avoid sensitisation to mouse gamma globulin. Patients were questioned closely as to their history of allergy to foreign protein or significant atopy. Such patients would be excluded from study but no such patient was submitted.

The large field of view gamma cameras (Siemens ZLC) is set up with a general purpose parallel hole collimator designed for energies up to 200 Kev for I-123 or Tc-99m; or designed for energies up to 300 Kev for In-111 studies. The gamma camera is peaked for the appropriate energies with a 20% window and for In-111 the counts in the two energy windows are summed. Uniformity and quality control is performed daily to ensure its optimal performance. The data are recorded on line to a Nodecrest Micas 3 computer for further image analysis.

The patient lies supine on the scanning couch and a gamma camera is placed over the pelvis anteriorly. The injection of 100-150 MBq (2.5 - 3.5 mCi) of I-123 labelled monoclonal antibody is given intravenously to the patient. Static images, each containing 800,000 counts are taken at 10 minutes, 4 hours & 22 hours anteriorly and posteriorly of the whole abdomen.

For each planar image, a similar image with radioactive Ba-133 markers over the prominent bony landmarks were taken to facilitate the subsequent repositioning of the patient (25). Similar procedures occur at 4 and 22 hours. For In-111 SM3, an injection of 80 - 120 MBg (2-3mCi) images were taken at ten min, 24, 48 or 72 hours. The final imaging was usually performed on the morning of surgery. For Tc-99m SM3 an injection of 600 MBq (15 mCi) was used and images were taken at 5 min, 3,6 & 22 hours. In each study between 0.5 and 1mg of monoclonal antibody was administered. All image data is transformed directly to the computer as well as to the microdot transparent film processor unit.

Radioimmunotherapy

Intracavity radioimmunotherapyfor cancer has been undertaken at this hospital since 1985. The criteria for entry into a trial of intraperitoneal therapy were those patients who had failed standard debulking surgery for stage III ovarian cancer, which was followed by full chemotherapy (30,31) and who, after a second or third look laparatomy, where further debulking of the tumour was undertaken, had residual deposits less than 2cm in size. These had to be confined to the peritoneal cavity and the liver had to be free of metastases. Renal function had to be adequate to enable the excretion of free ^{131}I. The antibody was usually HMFG2 or HMFG1.

In vitro studies on biopsies of the original tumour were undertaken to determine binding to HMFG1 or 2 as assessed by immunoperoxidestaining. Either radioimmunoscintigraphywith 123-I HMFG2 was performed 24 hours before the second look laparotomy to assess the specificity and the amount of uptake of HMFG2 into the tumour and/or 1mCi (40 MBq) 123-I HMFG2 in two litres of dialysis fluid was administered through a cannula. This was inserted into the peritoneal cavity under ultrasound control using a local anaesthetic. Gamma camera imaging was then used to assess the degree of uptake into the tumour.

The patient was prepared for therapy. The need for isolation during the treatment was explained as were the psychological problems of infrequent nursing attention, limited visiting and special disposable utensils and clothing. Potassium Iodide 120mg daily was started 2 days before and continued for 4 weeks after the therapy. Potassium perchlorate 400mg was given orally 30 minutes before the instillation of the unsealed source radioactive monoclonal antibody therapy.

The therapy dose in a lead shield vial was brought to the bedside. It was connected to the patient via a spinal needle inserted under the fluid level attached by an infusion extension line to a three way tap to the intra peritoneal cannula, Figure 1. A 10ml syringe containing saline was connected to the three way tap. With the tube to the therapy vial closed, 10 ml of saline is injected into the patient to check the patency of the cannula. A syringe containing 20ml saline is inserted into the top of the therapy vial. The three way tap is the opened to the vial and to the patient and saline is slowly injected into the therapy vial forcing the radiotherapy dose into the patient. The three way tap is then switched off in the direction of the patient. A 20ml syringe full of air is drawn up and inserted into the therapy vial. The three way tap is then opened to the vial and to the patient and the air injected into the therapy vial forcing the remaining liquid into the patient. The cannula is then removed and the site is checked to ensure the absence of leakage.

Using whole body counter measurements,the patient was then allowed home when the total body activity was less than 15mCi. The efficacy of radioimmunotherapywas assessed clinically, radiologically and by a further laparatomy 3 months later if there was no evidence of progressive disease.

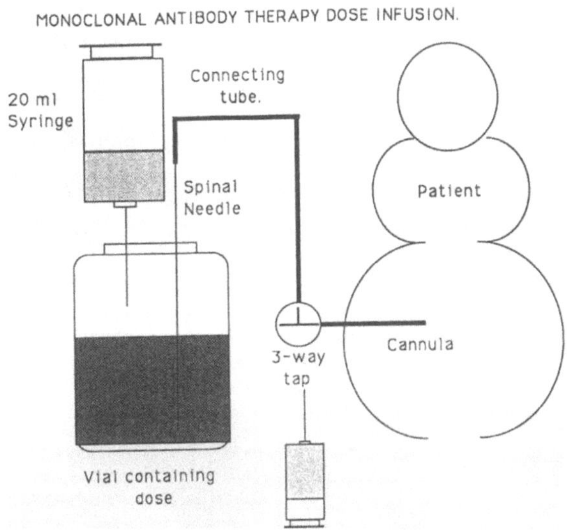

Fig.1 Diagram of the Infusion System for IntraperitonealRadioimmunotherapy.

Results of Radioimmunoscintigraphy with Radiolabelled SM3

The images from RIS were reported jointly by two nuclear medicine physicians in the absence of clinical and radiological information. The site of a primary tumour was described and for the serial changes in uptake, a decision as to whether it was benign or malignant was made. Specific uptake in a malignant tumour typically is low or absent on the 10 minute image and uptake increases with time. A benign vascular tumour such as a fibroid has a high initial non specific uptake decreasing with time as the blood activity falls. A benign cyst appears as a defect without a change in intensity in its wall whereas a malignant cyst shows increasing uptake peripherally with often some focal uptake. Recurrences may be identified at pelvic, paracolic, paraaortic, omental, hepatic or pulmonary sites. Malignant ascites typically shows a horseshoe of negative uptake in the 10 minute image, which has increased uptake with time, often with sites of focal uptake, for example in the omentum.

The results of RIS were compared with diagnostic radiological, surgical and histological findings. The largest series of patients were studied with In-111 SM3 : 29 using In-111 DTPA chelate and 6 using an In-111 9N3 macrocycle chelate (Celltec). Positive uptake was reported on RIS in the following benign ovarian tumours: some serious cystadenoma, a ruptured dermoid cyst, a mucinous cystadenoma and an ovarian fibroma. Where tested, SM3 uptake was shown on immunoperoxidise staining. Lack of uptake was noted in endometriosis. Uptake was also seen in some uterine leiomyoma and in cystic glandular endometrial hyperplasia. All but one malignant ovarian and uterine primary or recurrent tumour was reported correctly including serous papillary and mucinous cystadenocarcinomas, endometrioid and clear cell carcinomas, mixed mesodermal tumour, undifferentiated carcinoma, and endometrial carcinomas (Fig.2). One large cyst was called malignant but was benign on histology. This gave for In-111 SM3 an overall sensitivity for gynaecological malignancy of 96% but a specificity of only 33%, accuracy 75%. However the results using In-111 macrocycle SM3 were better with an accuracy of 83% compared to In-111 DTPA chelate SM3, accuracy of 69%.

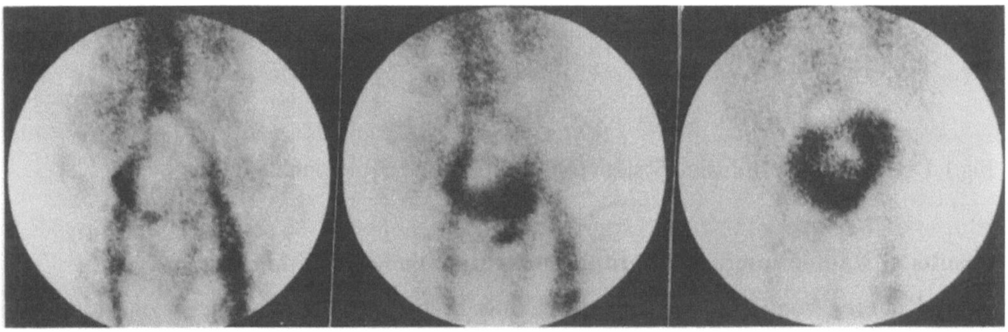

Fig 2 Ovarian adenocarcinomas imaged with Tc-99m SM3 monoclonal antibody Anteriour views of the pelvis: left, 10 minutes; centre, 6 hours; right 24 hours.

The results with I-123 SM3 gave a sensitivity of 100%, specificity of 67% and accuracy of 86% but with Tc-99m SM3 all the malignant and benign tumours were correctly identified, Table I.

Results of IntraperitonealRadioimmunotherapy

11 out of 18 patients assessed met the criteria for intraperitonealtherapy. The results were progressive disease in five, and in one, regressive at one site but progressive at another was confirmed at a third look laparotomy. Three patients progressed and died without undergoing laparotomy. One survived 13 months refusing operation and one showed a partial remission at laparotomy.

	111-In	123-I	99m-Tc	Total
Number of Studies	36*	7	12	55
Number of Patients	35	7	12	54
Positive Images	31	5	10	46
Malignant	23	4	10	37
Non Malignant	8	1	0	9
Negative Images	5	2	2	9
Malignant	1	0	0	1
Non Malignant	4	2	2	8
Sensitivity for Malignancy	96%	100%	100%	97%
Specificity for Malignancy	33%	67%	100%	47%
Accuracy for Malignancy	75%	86%	100%	82%

* 6 with 111-In macrocycle 9N3 [Celltec]

Table I. SM3 Radioimmunoscintigraphy in Pelvic Masses

The main complications were in the short term: depression due to isolation in the therapy room in one; dysphagia, severe in two and mild in one; and partial small bowel obstruction managed conservatively in two. In the longer term, two patients developed ileocutaneous fistulas. In one patient operated on 6 months after radioimmunotherapy,it was thought to be related to irradiation of malignant plaques on the small bowel wall, from the appearance of grossly irradiated tissue. Haematological complications were not severe. A transitory drop of all haematological indices to about 80% of pretreatment values was seen at 4-8 weeks. In one patient prolonged thrombocytopaeniawas seen (under 17 x $10^9 L^{-1}$) but not requiring platelet transfusion.

These results may be compared with those of Stewart at al (16). None of 9 patients with over 2cm diameter disease showed a beneficial response, 2/15 with less than 2cm diameter disease and 3/5 with microscopic disease showed partial remission. The results of Riva et al (31,33) using up to 150 mCi I-131 labelled monoclonal antibody with often serial doses are more encouraging. In 14 patients with ovarian cancer, one showed a complete remission (10 months so far), 2 a partial remission, 5 stabilisation of disease and 6 progression. It was noted that those with remission had the highest assessed tumour irradiation 7.5 Gy as compared to those with progression 2.5 Gy. It was noted the shorter the time since diagnosis in ovarian cancer, the more likely a remission after intraperitoneal radioimmunotherapy.

Such disappointing results led to a reassessment of the problems of intraperitoneal radioimmunotherapyfor ovarian cancer by Ward et al (34). A series of studies were undertaken just before second look laparotomy using the same antibody, HMFG2, labelled with different radionuclides to compare intravenous with intraperitoneal administration. Examination and counting of tissue obtained at surgery showed that many ovarian 'peritoneal' metastases were, in fact, sub-serosal and received a greater amount of the injected activity from the intravenous than from the intraperitonealinjection, whereas the truly intraperitonealtumour received more from the intraperitonealthan the intravenous injection. Malignant cells in ascites, in particular, took up as much as 70 times more antibody from the intraperitoneal than the intravenous injection.

The second study compared simultaneous intraperitoneal administration of the specific tumour-associated antibody with a non-specific antibody, each with a different radiolabel. Surgical excision of metastases showed, a wide range of heterogeneity of uptake by solid tumour with localisation ranging from equal specific and non-specific uptake at one site to a 4 to 100 times uptake by the specific over the non-specific antibody. Excellent uptake of specific antibody was seen in malignant cells in ascitic fluid. The localisation index which is the ratio of tumour to normal tissue uptake for the specific antibody divided by the ratio of tumour to normal tissue uptake for the non-specific antibody gave values of between one to one and four to one for solid tumours over 7 days, but eleven to one for malignant ascites cells.

After intraperitoneal injection the radio-iodine label was cleared from the body approximately exponentially with a half life of 18 hours. Over 80% of the intraperitoneally injected radioactivity was found as non-protein bound iodine in the urine by 7 days. Such urinary excretion helps to reduce the irradiation of normal tissues, but a high fluid intake and frequent bladder emptying are required to reduce the dose absorbed to the local bladder wall.

The successful documentation of therapeutically sufficient uptakes of radiolabelled monoclonal antibody by malignant cells in ascitic fluid has been followed by a pilot study. Five patients with malignant ascites (two colonic adenocarcinoma, two ovarian adenocarcinoma and one peritoneal papillary mesothelioma) were treated with between 75 and 150 mCi (3-6 GBq) of ^{131}I-labelled selective antibody. This was AUA1 antibody against a small glycoprotein antigen expressed in gastrointestinal adenocarcinomas for the colonic cancers and HMFG2 for the others (31). One patient lost his massive ascites completely, dying of recurrent abdominal solid tumour after 4 months without further ascites. The second was in extremis and died shortly after treatment but his ascetic fluid was shown to be clear of malignant cells. The third patient had recurrent malignant ascites but was free of HMFG2 binding ovarian cancer cells against which therapy was targeted. The fourth and fifth were free of ascites for 4 months before recurrence, much longer than to be expected from repeated tapping. The question remains however: how do these results compare with the former intraperitoneal therapy with colloidal gold, ^{198}Au whose uptake was non-specific. To this end a randomised prospective multicentre study of ^{131}I-labelled appropriate specific or ^{131}I-labelled non-specific antibody at an administered dose of about 100mCi (4GBq) in malignant pleural effusion or ascites has been instituted. Over twenty patients have been included but the code has not yet broken, so the outcome is not evaluated.

An alternative approach to solid intraperitoneal tumour is needed. As well as the lack of delivery of an adequate therapeutic dose due to the low percentage uptake of the administered radiolabelled antibody there is the great heterogeneity of uptake by metastatic or recurrent diseases. It has been argued that the use of a higher energy, longer range Beta emitter would kill malignant cells not expressing the antigen that were adjacent to those taking up the antibody. Yttrium 90 (^{90}Y) is such a radionuclide (64 h half-life) with a maximum Beta energy of 2.2 MeV giving a potential crossfire range of 11mm. It is a metal and is labelled to antibody using a chelating agent, the cyclic anhydride of diethylene triamine penta-acetate (DTPA), by the technique of Hnatowich et al.(35).However, our in vitro studies have shown that the binding of ^{90}Y to antibody is relatively weak and cannot easily be optimized (36). That the escape of free ^{90}Y is rapid from intraperitoneally administered ^{90}Y-labelled antibody is demonstrated by two studies of one patient with malignant ascites due to ovarian cancer. In the first, given 10mCi (0.40 GBq), the maximum blood activity was 10%, obtained at 20 h, and changed little. In contrast, in the second administration, given 12mCi (0.48 GBq), a chelating agent, ethylene diamene tetra-acetate (EDTA) was infused intravenously causing the peak plasma level at 20 h to fall rapidly. The large amount circulating free ^{90}Y targets to bone and accounts for the high marrow toxicity seen with 12-20 mCi (0.48-0.8 GBq) of ^{90}Y-labelled antibody reported by Stewart et al (16). ^{90}Y will not be satisfactory for intraperitoneal radioimmunotherapy until a better, more stable chelating system is available such as the appropriate macrocyclic compound together with a method of promoting the excretion of radioactive ^{90}Y metabolites from the blood stream.

Discussion and Conclusion

In radioimmunoscintigraphy of gynaecological malignancy the move from In-123 to Tc-99m as the radiolabel appears to be justified. From preliminary results, it also appears that use of an In-111 macrocycle is preferable to the cyclic anhydride of DTPA as the chelating agent. In spite of the theory, no important difference between SM3 and HMFG1 has been shown in the differentiation of benign serous and mucinous cystadenoma from malignant. It remains to be determined whether OVTL3 is more specific although initial results are encouraging (20). The importance of this distinction is the urgent need to reduce the number of unnecessary operations on well women whose pelvic ultrasound has found a mass. 5000 screened, 324 operated and only 9 ovarian cancers were found (5). Interpolation of RIS with a specific antibody which does not react with benign ovarian or uterine masses or with pelvic inflammatory disease between positive ultrasound and the decision to operate should increase the percentage of 'necessary operations'. Many unanswered questions remain. Should ovarian cystadenomas be considered premalignant? Most pathologists argue not. Should they be removed anyhow? What is the outcome if they remain? Should every simple cyst be removed? What is the chance of rupture?. The combination of ultrasound and more specific RIS with the Tc-99m label giving a low absorbed radiation dose may help to answer these questions, if applied serially to those in whom operation may be considered unnecessary.

The improvement in the antibody from humanisation through recombinant DNA techniques and CRD grafting (37) and through the change from the hybridoma approach to the bacterial bioengineer using genetic engineering and the polymerase chain reaction (38) will reduce the HAMA response. This is of little benefit in diagnostic work (39) but important for therapy. Genetic engineering also allows the development of small active binding molecules, the single domain antibody 'dAbs' where the active site of the heavy V_H chain is arranged at one end of the peptide with the combining site of the light V_L chain at the other, yet it still retained immunoreactivity (40). The uses of bifunctional antibodies such as Fv_1-Fv_2 where Fv_1 reacts with the cancer antigen and Fv_2 with the diagnostic or therapy radionuclide will have the advantages of allowing tumour penetration and clearance of the unlabelled antibody in a two stage or three stage approach (41). The use of lambda phage approach to genetic engineering gives the potential of unlimited development of and rapid screening for specific antibody Fv fragments (42). The oncogene-antioncogene-protooncogene theory of cancer (43) indicates that there are genetic differences in the malignant cell from its normal counterpart. These are related to segments of DNA encoding expressor or suppressor genes. Oncogene amplification correlates with the degree of malignancy (44). For such active DNA segments in cancer there are equivalent RNA and thus amino acid sequences generating the effector or suppressor oncoproteins. By choice of oncoproteins representing the malignant process and development of monoclonal antibodies against these, cancer specificity may be obtainable. This has already been demonstrated for the c-myc oncogene in lung cancer imaged using an antioncoprotein monoclonal antibody (43). Once such cancer specific antibodies are identified, development of genetically engineered humanised bispecific antibodies should follow.

The intracavity approach is used in the hope that a larger radiation dose will be delivered to the local tumour tissues than the normal critical tissue. Since the radiolabelled antibody or its radioactive breakdown products diffuse rather rapidly into the normal body tissues with a half time of about a day, the use of high energy, short lived radionuclides for therapy such as Re-186 (T1/2 3.8 days, Beta 1.07 MeV) as a Tc-99m substitute, Cu-67 (T1/2 2.4 days, Beta

0.45-0.57), Sm-153 (T1/2 2 days, Beta 0.64-0.81), and Y-90 (T1/2 2.7 days, Beta 2.27 MeV) are advocated (45). Thus by the time of diffusion into the normal tissues, much of the activity will have decayed.

There is an alternative scenario. Let the normal tissues be completely cleared by chasing the antibody out of the circulation to liver or kidneys after the antibody has been bound to the tumour, as Goodwin (46) has frequently advocated. If the level of radiolabelled antibody not in the tumour could be reduced towards zero, then a new perspective of long lived resident radioimmunotherapycould be addressed. Radionuclides such as P32 (T1/2 14.3 days, Beta 1.7 MeV), In-114m (T1/2 60 days, Beta 2.0 MeV), I-125 (T1/2 60 days, auger electrons) could be used and the tumouricidal radiation dose would be due to the area under the activity residence time curve, where the long irradiation time makes up for the relatively low tumour uptake of the antibody as a percentage of the injected dose.

Long lived therapy is effective as seen with I-131 T1/2 8 days, Beta 1.61 MeV) for thyroid cancer (47), and with Sr-89 (T1/2 50.5 days, Beta 1.5 MeV) for palliation of pain of prostatic cancer where pain relief may last for six months (48), and with In-114m (T1/2 60 days, Bate 2 MeV) labelled lymphocytes for Hodgkins Disease (49). In-114m would fit in nicely into the recently developed macrocycles for binding Indium (11) to radiolabelled antibodies. P32 may be bound by the simple Kemptide sequence of amino acids (50) which may be incorporated into an antibody, chemically or by genetic engineering, to give a stable P32 labelled antibody (17).

One approach to a clearance technique is to use a bifunctional antibody one end reacting with the cancer and the other with a radioactive therapy containing ligand (51). These may be developed using the quadroma technique or though genetic engineering particularly the Fv-Fv approach. Injection of the bifunctional antibody, preferably labelled with a simple radiotracer such as Tc-99m using the modified Schwarz method (14) would confirm tumour uptake and allow determination of the rate of tissue clearance to liver or kidney over the next 24 hours. In this way the optimum time for injection of the radiotherapy-labelled ligand would be determined. A modification of this approach is to use the high binding affinity of Streptavidin for biotin. Either biotinylated antibody followed by Streptavidin attached radiotherapy or vice versa could be used (52,53,54). although early experience has not been so encouraging (55).

A three stage approach may be considered (56). First the smallest molecule should be used for tumour penetration therefore biotin-antibody fragment (humanised, genetically engineered,

Fv etc.) but labelled with In-111 to track and confirm its uptake. Then the Streptavidin alone to clear the blood and tissues of the Biotin antibody fragment. Again a radiolabel such as Tc-99m would allow the clearance process to be followed. Then the Biotinylated long lived radiotherapy bearing ligand would follow and target to the tumour and deposit, preferably through internalisation, its radioactive bullet (I-125, P32 or In-114m etc.) to provide the long lived resident radioimmunotherapysupported by an unimpeded immunological response in a body receiving minimal irradiation of the normal critical tissues. That approach or a similar 2 or 3-stage approach using bifunctional antibodies hold the promise of successful radioimmunotherapy.

In conclusion, intracavityradioimmunotherapyhas been less successful than expected, except for its benefits in malignant meningitis (57,58). A two stage or three stage approach may be the only way of improving the therapeutic ratio by reducing the exposure of the normal critical tissues. This would then enable long lived radionuclides to be used for resident radioimmunotherapy, whereby the longer residence time would compensate for the relatively poor uptake that is the main problem of radioimmunotherapy. Meanwhile radioimmunoscintigraphy of ovarian cancer with Tc-99m as label has become a routine diagnostic procedure.

Acknowledgements

We are grateful for the support of the Imperial Cancer Research Fund and for the use of the facilities provided by the St. Bartholomew's Hospital Research Trust.

References

1. Granowska M, Britton K.E, Shepherd J.H, Nimmon C.C, Mather S, Ward B, Osborne R.J, Slevin M.L. [1986]. A prospective study of 123I-labelled monoclonal antibody imaging in ovarian cancer. J Clin Oncol. 4:730-6.

2. Granowska M, Shepherd J, Britton K.E, Ward B, Mather S, Taylor-Papadimitriou J, Epenetos A.A, Carroll M.J, Nimmon C.C, Hawkins L.A, Flatman W.D, Horne T, Bodmer W.F. [1984]. Ovarian cancer: diagnosis using I-123 monoclonal antibody in comparison with surgical findings. Nucl Med Commun. 5:485-499.

3. Chatal J.C, Fumoleau P, Saccavini J, Thedrez P, Curtet C, Bianco Arco A, Chetanneau A, Peltier P, Kremmer M, Guillard Y. [1987]. Immunoscintigraphy of recurrences of gynaecologic carcinomas.

4. Pateisky N, Philipp K, Skodler W.D, Czevwenka K, Hamilton G, Burchell J. [1985]. Radioimmunodetection in patients with suspected ovarian cancer. J. Nucl Med 26:1369-1376.

5. Campbell S, Bhan V, Royston P, Whitehead M.I, Collins W.P. [1989]. Transabdominal ultrasound screening for early ovarian cancer. Brit.Med. J. 229:1363-1367.

6. Epenetos A.A, Britton K.E, Mather S, Shepherd J, Granowska M, Taylor-Papadimitriou J, Nimmon C.C, Durbin H, Hawkins L.A, Malpas J.S, Bodmer W.F. [1982]. Targeting of Iodine-123 labelled tumour associated monoclonal antibodies to ovarian, breast and gastrointestinal tumours. Lancet ii, 999-1005.

7. Peltier P, Fumoleau P, Kremer M, Thedrez P, Chetanneau A, Chatal J.F. [1989]. Immunoscintigraphy of ovarian cancers using In-111-DTPA-OC125 monoclonal antibody. In: JF Chatal Ed Monoclonal antibodies in immunoscintigraphy. CRS Press. Boca Raton, Florida: 187-209.

8. Baum R.P, Hertel A, Lorenz M, Schwarz A, Encke A, Hor G. [1989]. Tc-99m labelled anti CEA monoclonal antibody for tumour immunoscintigraphy first clinical results. Nucl. Med. Commun. 10:345-348.

9. Granowska M, Jobling T, Britton K.E, Mather S.J, Naeem M. Shepherd J.H. [1990].
Tc-99m labelled monoclonal antibodies for radioimmunoscintigraphy of ovarian cancer, in H.A.E Schmidt and J.Chambron [eds] proc. Europ. Asoc. Nucl. Med. Cong. Strasbourg. Schattauer Stuttgart, in press.

10. Hnatowich D.J, Layne W.W, Childs R.L. [1983]. Radioactive labeling of antibody: a simple and effective method. Science; 220:613-615.

11. Cole W.C, DeNardo S.J, Meares C.F, McCall M.J, DeNardo G, Epstein A.L, O'Brien H.A, Moi M.K. [1987]. Comparative Serum stability of Radiochelates for Antibody Radiopharmaceuticals. J. Nucl. Med. 28:83-90.

12. Meares C.F, [1986]. Chelating agents for the binding of metal ions to antibodies. Nucl. Med. Biol. 13:311-318.

13. Rhodes B.A, Towestad D.A, Breslow K. [1983]. Tc-99m labelling and acceptance testing of radiolabelled antibodies and antibody fragments. In: Burchiel S.W, Rhodes B.A, [eds]. Radioimmunoimaging and radioimmunotherapy. New York: Elsevier Publishing Co, Inc. 111- 123.

14. Schwarz A, Steinstraesser A. [1987]. A novel approach to Tc-99m labelled monoclonal antibodies. J. Nucl. Med. 28:721.

15. Mather S.J, Ellison D. [1990]. Reduction medicated Technetium 99m labelling of monoclonal antibodies. J. Nucl. Med. in press.

16. Stewart J.S.W, Hird V, Sullivan M, Snook D, Epenetos A. [1989]. Intraperitoneal radioimmunotherapy for ovarian cancer. Brit. J. Obs. Gynaecol. 86:529-536.

17. Foxwell B.M.J, Band H.A, Long J, Jeffrey W.A, Snook D, Thorpe P.E, Watson G, Parker P.J, Epenetos A.A, Creighton A.M. [1988]. Conjugation of monoclonal antibodies to a synthetic peptide substrate for protein kinase: a method of labelling antibodies with 32-P. Brit. J. Cancer. 57:389-403.

18. Taylor-Papadimitriou J, Peterson J, Arklie J, Burchell J, Ceriani R.L, Bodmer W.F. [1981]. Monoclonal antibodies to epithelium specific components of the human milk fat globule membrane: production and reaction with cells in culture. Int. J. Cancer. 28:17-21.

19. Burchell J, Gendler S, Taylor-Papadimitriou J. [1987]. Development and characterization of breast cancer reactive monoclonal antibodies directed to the core protein of the human milk mucin. Cancer Res; 47:5476-5482.

20. Buist M.R, Roos J.C, Golding R.P, Burger C.W, Vermoreen J.B, Lingen A.V, Baak J.P.A, Hilgers J, Kenemans P. [1990]. Comparison of Immunoscintigraphy [111-In-OVTL3- F[ab]^2 with other diagnostic methods in the detection of tumour deposits in ovarian carcinoma patients. Antibody. Immunoconj. Radiopharm. 3:41.

21. Burchell J, Taylor-Papadimitriou J, Boshell M. [1989]. A short sequence, within the amino acid tendem repeat of a cancer-associated mucin, contains immunodominant epitopes. Int. J. Cancer; 44:4486-54.

22. Granowska M, Mather S.J, Jobling T, Naeem M, Burchell J, Taylor-Papadimitriou J, Shepherd J, Britton K.E. [1990]. Radiolabelled Stripped Mucin, SM3, Monoclonal Antibody for Immunoscintigraphy of Ovarian Tumours. Int. J. Biol. Mark. in press.

23. Goldenberg D.M, Kim E.E, Deland F.H, Benne H.S, Primus F,J. [1980]. Radioimmunodetection of cancer with radioactive antibodies to carcinoembryonic antigen. Cancer. Res. 40:2984-2992.

24. Ott R.J, Grey L.J, Zivanovic M.A, Flower M.A, Trott N.G, Moshakis V, Coombes R.C, Neville A.M, Ormerod M.G, Westwood J.H. [1983]. The limitations of the dual radionuclide subtraction technique for the external detection of tumours by radioiodine labelled antibodies. Brit. J. Radiol. 56:101-108.

25. Granowska M, Britton K.E, Shepherd J. [1984]. The detection of ovarian cancer using 1223-1 monoclonal antibody. Radiobiol. Radiother. [Berlin]; 25:153-160.

26. Granowska M, Nimmon C.C, Britton K.E, Mather S.J, Crowther M, Slevin M.L, Shepherd J.H. [1988]. Kinetic analysis and probability mapping applied to the detection of ovarian cancer by radioimmunoscintigraphy. J. Nucl. Med. 29:599-607.

27. Begent R.H.J. [1986]. Working party on the clinical use of antibodies: operations manual. Brit. J. Canc; 54:557-68.

28. Hnatowich D.J, Virzi F, Doherty P.W. [1985]. DTPA coupled antibodies labelled with Yttriun 90. J. Nucl. Med. 26:503-509.

29. Mather S.J, Ward B. [1987]. High efficiency iodination of monoclonal antibodies for radiol. J. Nucl. Med. 28:1034-7 30.

30. Crowther M.E, Ward B.G, Granowska M, Mather S, Britton K.E, Shepherd J.H, Slevin M.L. [1989]. Therapeutic considerations in the use of intra-peritoneal radiolabelled monoclonal antibodies in ovarian carcinoma. Nucl. Med. Commun. 10:384-388.

31. Ward B, Mather S, Shepherd J, Crowther M, Hawkins L, Britton K, Slevin M.L. [1988] The treatment of intraperitoneal malignant disease with monoclonal antibody guided 131-I radiotherapy. Brit. J. Cancer. 58:658-662.

32. Riva p, Marangolo M, Lazzari S, Moscatelli G, Sarti G, Agostini M, Spinelli A, Franceschi G, Gasperoni R, Tirindelli D. [1989] Locoregional and systemic administration of radiolabelled monoclonal antibodies in solid tumour treatment: a phase I study. Reg. Cancer Treat 1. 164-169.

33. Riva P, Lazzari S, Tison V, Armaroli L, Franceschi G, Moscatelli G, Sarti G, Spinelli A, Morigi P, Vecchietti G, Mazzotti C, Tirindelli D. [1990]. Therapeutic applications of radiolabelled monoclonal antibodies in gastrointestinal and ovarian tumours: analysis of the anatomical, biological, clinical, and physical parameters which influence the response to Radioimmunotherapy. In Radioisotopes in Clinical Research and Practice. Hofer R, Bergmann H [eds] Vienna, in press.

34. Ward B.G, Mather S.J, Hawkins L.A, Crowther M.E, Shepherd J.H, Granowska M, Britton K.E, Slevin M.L. [1987]. Localisation of Radioiodine conjugated to monoclonal antibody HMFG2 in human ovarian carcinoma: assessment of intravenous and intraperitoneal ratios of administration. Cancer. Res. 47:4719-4723.

35. Hnatowich D.J, Virzi F, Doherty P.W. [1985]. DTPA coupled antibodies labelled with Yttrium-90. J. Nucl. Med. 26:503-509.

36. Mather S.J, Tolley D. [1988]. Labelling of monoclonal antibodies with 90-Y. Nucl.Med. Commun. 9:182-183.

37. Reichmann L, Clark M, Waldmann H, Winter G. [1988]. Reshaping human antibodies for therapy. Nature, 332, 323-327.

38. Rodwell J.D. [1989]. Engineering monoclonal antibodies. Nature, 342, 99-100.

39. Baum R.P, Hertel A, Madry N, Chatenoud L, Reynolds J.C, Saccavini J.C, Auerbach B, Larson S.M, Hor G. [1988]. Human antimouse antibody [HAMA] response: short and long term follow up in 76 patients after diagnostic and therapeutic application of radiolabelled monoclonal antibodies. In Nuklearmedizin, Proc 25th Cong Soc Nucl Med Europe Budapest 1987. Schmidt H.A.E, Csernay L. [eds]. Schattauer, Stuttgart 608-610.

40. Ward E.S, Gussow D, Griffiths A.D, Jones P.T, Winter G. [1989], Binding activities of a repertoire of single immunoglobulin variable domains from Escherichia coli. Nature, 341, 544- 546.

41. Britton K.E. [1990]. Overview of Radioimmunotherapy. Proc. 5th int. Conf. Monoclonal Antibody Immunoconjugates for Cancer. Antibody Immunoconj. Radiopharm. 3, in press.

42. Huse W,D. Sastry L, Iversan S.A, Karg A.S, Alting-Mees M, Burton D,R. Benkovik, S.J, Lerner R.A. [1990].Generation of a large combinatorial library of the Immunoglobulin repertoire in phage Lambden. Science 246, 1275-1281.

43. Chan S, Sikora K. [1987]. The potential of oncogene products as tumour markers. Cancer Surveys 6, 185-207.

44. Schrab M, Alitalo K, Klempnauer K.B, Varmus H.E, Bishop J.M, Gelbert E, Brodeur G, Goldstein M, Trent J. [1983]. Amplified DNA with limited homology to myc cellular oncogene is shared by human neuroblastoma cell lines and a neuroblastoma tumour. Nature 305, 245-248.

45. Britton K.E, Slevin M.L, Mather S.J, Crowther M, Ward B, Granowska M, Naeem M, Ellison D, Hawkins L.A, Shepherd J. [1990]. Radiolabelled antibodies in therapy. In Monoclonal antibodies and Immunoconjugates in cancer treatment. Parthenon, Cornforth, in press.

46. Goodwin D.A, Mears C.F, McCall M.J, McTigue M, Chaovapong W. [1988]. Pretargetted Immunoscintigraphy of murine tumours with In-111 labelled bifunctional haptens. J. Nucl. Med. 29:226-234.

47. Beierwaltes W.H. [1976]. The treatment of thyroid carcinoma with radioactive iodine. Sem. Nucl. Med. 8:79-94.

48. Blake G.M, Gray J.M, Zivanovic M.A, McEwan A.J, Fleming J.S, Ackery D.M. [1987]. Strontium-89 radionuclide therapy: a dosimetric study using impulse response function analysis. Brit. J. Radiol. 60:685-692.

49. Hamilton D, Cowan R.A, Drayson M, Sharma K, Cummins P.E.C, Nuttall P.M, Deakin D, Wagstaff J, Crowther D. [1988]. 114-In-m Oxine-labelled lymphocytes - therapeutic applications. Nucl. Med. Commun. 9:797-802.

50. Kemp B.E, Graves D.J, Benjamin E. [1976]. Synthetic Peptide subtrates of the cAMP- dependent protein kinase. Fed. Proc. 35, 1384.

51. Goodwin D.A, Meares C.F, McCall M.J, Chaovapong W, McTigue M, Diamanti C.I. [1989]. Improved tumour uptake with In-111, Ga-67 and Ga-68 labelled bivalent heptans in pretargetted immunoscintigraphy. J. Nucl. Med. 30:762.

52. Goodwin D.A, Meares C.F, McCall M.J, McTigue M, Chaovapong W. [1987]. An avidin biotin chelate system for imaging tumours. J. Nucl. Med. 28:722.

53. Pimm M.V, Fells H.F, Perkins A.C, Baldwin R.W. [1988]. Iodine 131 and Indium-111 labelled avidin and streptavidin for pretargetted immunoscintigraphy with biotinylated anti- tumour monoclonal antibody. Nucl. Med. Commun. 11:931-941.

54. Paganelli G, Riva P, Deleide G, Clivco A, Cholerio F, Scassellati G.A, Malcovati M, Siccardi A.G. [1989]. Targeting of biotinylated anti-tumour monoclonal antibodies by means of radioactive avidin or streptavidin in an animal model. Nucl. Med. Biol. 16:177-178.

55. Kalofonos H.P, Rusckowski M, Lavender J.P, Epenetos A.A, Hnatowich D.J. [1989]. Radioimmunotargeting of tumour in patients with Streptavidin and Biotin. J. Nucl. Med. 30:819.

56. Britton K.E. [1989]. In Fazio F, and Paganelli G, proceedings of a workshop in Streptanidin Butin linkage of monoclonal antibodies. Milan, in preparation.

57. Coakham H.B, Richardson R.B, Davies A.G, Bourne S.P, Eckert H, Kemshead J.T. [1988]. Neoplastic meningitis from a pineal tumour treated by antibody guided irradiation via the intrathecal route. Brit. J. Neurosurg. 2:199-209.

58. Coakham H.B, Wheeler J. [1989]. Immunolocalisation of cerebral tumours. Rad. 15, 29-33.

MONOCLONAL ANTIBODIES FOR CELL LABELLING WITH PARTICULAR REFERENCE TO THROMBUS IMAGING

A.C. Perkins and R.J. Lonsdale

Abstract

Advances in biotechnology have resulted in a range of monoclonal antibodies directed against circulating blood cells and serum proteins, with antibodies against granulocytes being used for the detection of inflammation and localised infection and antibodies specific for platelets and fibrin being used for imaging thrombi. The use of monoclonal antibodies for cell labelling represents one of the most exciting of the recent developments in nuclear medicine and offers the potential for revolutionising current radiopharmacy practice.

Clinical studies with the platelet specific antibody P256 Fab' carried out at the Hammersmith Hospital in London and at University Hospital in Nottingham have demonstrated the successful imaging of venous and arterial thrombi and pulmonary embolism. The use of this antibody for the detection and characterisation of arterial thrombi in patients being considered for thrombolytic therapy would appear to be particularly promising. These studies demonstrate the clinical impact that these agents are potentially capable of producing.

Introduction

The continued development of monoclonal antibodies associated with tumour antigens has led to the assumption that radiolabelled antibodies are firmly linked with the diagnosis and therapy of cancer. However, developments taking place during the late 1980s have resulted in the application of monoclonal antibodies for the investigation of benign conditions. Much of the early work with monoclonal antibodies concentrated on the search for antigens specific for tumours with the ultimate goal being the delivery of cytotoxic agents for tumour therapy. Whilst the application of monoclonal antibodies for tumour therapy has been limited, their use had become routinely accepted in some quarters for the diagnosis of malignant disease and in particular the monitoring of tumour response to treatment. The number of antibodies which are available for clinical application is steadily growing and although initially discarded because

R. P. Baum et al. (eds.), Clinical Use of Antibodies, 111–120.

of their poor tumour targeting properties, antibodies reacting specifically with some normal tissues are now realising potential as agents for the selective labelling of specific cells, cellular components and circulating proteins.

Clinical studies with these materials are now under way both in the United States and Europe and it is already evident that antibodies offer a number of advantages for cell labelling compared with conventional techniques. Previous cell labelling techniques have involved time consuming procedures on blood samples, such as cell separation, incubation, resuspension and washing. Using an appropriate antibody, cells may be radiolabelled invivo following a single intravenous injection, thus eliminating the demand on time and facilities within the radiopharmacy. Two main categories of monoclonal antibody have been developed and used clinically, these being antibodies against granulocytes and those reacting with platelets and fibrin.

Antibodies reacting with granulocytes and leucocytes

Imaging localised collections of radiolabelled leucocytes is now an established and reliable technique for the detection of abscess and inflammatory processes and has now largely replaced the more traditional use of Ga-67 gallium citrate. The choice of agents available for this application has expanded considerably over recent years and the technique of choice remains to be proven. A list of the radio-pharmaceuticals currently available for imaging sites of inflammation or infection is given in Table 1, The most common procedure currently used involves radiolabelling the patients own leucocytes with In-111 indium oxine or Tc-99m hexamethylpropyleneamineoxime(HMPAO) prior to reinjection (Danpure et al 1985, Peters et al 1986),

Table 1 Radiopharmaceuticals available for the detection of abscess and inflammation

Ga-67 gallium citrate

In-111 indium oxine-labelled leucocytes

Tc-99m HMPAO-labelled leucocytes

I-123/Tc-99m anti-granulocte antibody

Tc-99m/In111 Polyclonal human immunogloblulin (HIG)

For the detection of abscess it may be ultimately desirable to use antibodies reactive with specific microbial antigens, however such antibodies are not yet available. Currently available anti-granulocyteantibodies are less specific since they localise at sites of both inflammation and infection. The use of these agents has largely resulted from the identification of antibodies which were originally raised against CEA but, subsequently found to react with the 95 KiloDalton non-specificcross reacting antigen NCA-95. Antibodies such as A-47 (Granuloscint) and BW 250/183 (Granulozyt) have been used with either Tc-99m, I-123 or In-111 as the radiolabel (Locher et al 1986, Joseph et al 1988). Clinical studies include the detection and localisation of sites of bone infection, inflammation bowel disease, pancreatitis and bone marrow imaging.

A number of antibodies have now been raised specifically against neutrophils, however further clinical work will be necessary to assess the value of these materials (Thakur et al 1988). Overall the clinical value of these agents will need to be assessed in comparison with the more established cell labelling procedures and the more recently introduced polyclonal human immunoglobulin (HIG)

Antibodies reacting with platelets and fibrin

Platelet labelling using In-111 indium oxine has been available since 1978 (Hawkes et al). This technique was largely developed as a research tool for the assessment of platelet deposition in experimental coronary artery bypass angioplasty and vascular surgery. The technique is limited, requiring a more accurate and time consuming separation of cells than for the labelling of leucocytes. Administered doses are generally low being less than 40 MBq, resulting in poor quality images containing low count rates. Monoclonal antibodies reacting with antigens associated with thrombus formation are now becoming available. In general these antibodies react with the 11b/111a glycoprotein platelet cell membrane receptor, activated platelet antigens and the amino terminus of fibrin 11 (see Table 2).

7E3 and 10E5 antibodies

Antibodies 7E3 and 10E3 both reactive with the 11b/111a receptor (the fibrinogen binding site on the platelet cell surface) were developed by Coller et al 1981. These antibodies in both intact and F(ab')2 form were shown to completely block platelet aggregation induced by ADP and to partially inhibit platelet aggregation induced by collagen and thrombin. The earliest

TABLE 2 ANTIBODIES FOR THROMBUS IMAGING (Characterised by target epitope)

Platelet specific		Fibrin specific
11b/111a Receptor	**Activated platelet Antigens**	**Amino Terminus of Fibrin 11**
P256	anti-GM140	64C5
7E3	S12	59D8
10E3	TSP/TSP 1.1	T2G1s
50H.19		DD-3B6-22
B59.2		GC4
PAC-1		

report of successful thrombus imaging with a monoclonal antibody was published in 1985 by Oster et al. This work was carried out in an animal model and cell labelling was achieved by incubating autologous blood with In-111-7E3 prior to reinjection. Despite these initial results the properties of inhibiting platelet aggregation have meant that this antibody was more suitable for therapy where it has been used as an adjuvant to coronary artery thrombosis (Gold et al 1988).

P256 platelet specific antibody

Unlike other antibodies which have been developed for thrombus imaging the monoclonal antibody P256 originally produced in the UK by the Imperial Cancer Research Fund has been used in a number of clinical trials. Whereas the 7E3 antibody was raised against platelets the P256 antibody was raised by the immunisation of mice with human monocytes. Initial studies with this antibody were carried out at the Hammersmith Hospital in London leading to published studies demonstrating the successful imaging of deep vein thrombosis and pulmonary embolism (Peters et al 1986, Stuttle et al 1988a, 1989), Contrary to the findings using 7E3 antibody, use of the P256 antibody in intact and bivalent form resulted in platelet aggregation invitro (Stuttle et al 1988b). Consequently, clinical use of the Fab' fragment of this antibody has been advocated.

The Nottingham P256 studies

Studies initiated at Nottingham have examined the capabilities of the P256 Fab' for the assessment of arterial thrombi. This work has included the detection and characterisation of peripheral arterial thromboses prior to thrombolytic therapy and monitoring platelet deposition following angioplasty. Intra-arterial thrombosis has become established as an important method of treating selected arterial occlusions. The aim of our studies was to assess the clinical value of immunoscintigraphy using platelet arterial occlusion. Thrombolytic agents such as Streptokinase and Tissue Plasminogen Activator are highly effective in achieving recanalisation of recent thrombotic arterial occlusions, thereby avoiding amputation or surgical reconstruction but, are much less effective in treating chronic occlusions. Arteriography does not reliably distinguish between acute and chronic arterial occlusions and it does not select the patients whom are most likely to benefit from thrombolytic therapy. Attempted thrombolysis of chronic lesions unnecessarily exposes patients to the recognised risks of bleeding and stroke (Berridge et al 1989). Current knowledge indicates that arterial thrombi are rich in platelets and low in fibrin. Platelet specific antibodies should therefore be more suitable for imaging arterial thrombi.

Our initial results demonstrated that radiolabelling of the P256 Fab' antibody using In-111 produced greater than 95% incorporation of the radiolabel, with approximately 80% of blood-borne activity associated with the platelet fraction (Frier et al 1990). Twenty patients with acute peripheral lower limb ischaemia were investigated following the intravenous administrations of 100μg P256 Fab' radiolabelled with 20MBq In-111. Anterior and posterior views were recorded at 20 min, 2-5 hours and 24 hours after administration using a gamma camera fitted with a medium energy collimator (300keV maximum energy). Thirteen of these patients subsequently underwent arteriography and thrombolysis using Streptokinase or TPA.

Images of high quality were obtained as early as 4 hours following administration. The image appearances fell into one of three main types: focal increased uptake, diffuse increased uptake and no increased uptake. Fig.1 shows an example of focal uptake in a patient with thrombi in the left superficial femoral artery. Chronic occlusions thought on clinical grounds to be of greater than 30 days duration were not visualised. Of the 13 patients in whom thrombolysis was attempted, six patients had positive uptake of antibody at the site of thrombi, All six patients underwent successful lysis and this was maintained in four patients. Of the other 7 patients with negative images, 5 had either immediate rethrombosis following therapy or failed lysis and the remaining 2 patients lysed successfully. In a further series of patients P256 Fab' antibody has been used to demonstrate the reformation of thrombi following balloon angioplasty. An example of a patient with extensive uptake in the right superficial femoral artery is shown in Fig.2.

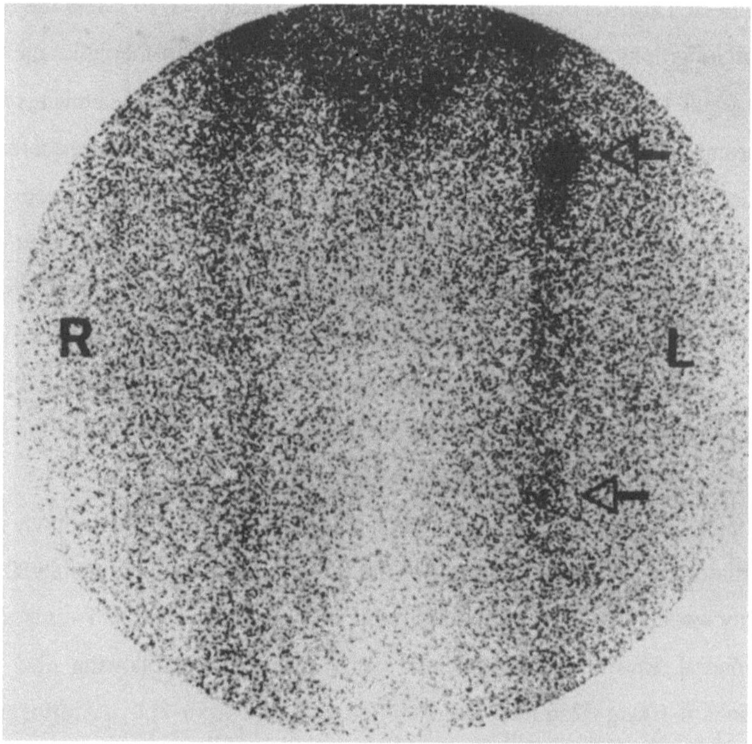

Figure 1. Anterior views of the thigh region of a patient with arterial thrombi in the left superficial femoral artery following administration of In-111 P256 Fab' antibody. Two sites of focal increased uptake (arrows) can be seen with a line of increased uptake between these sites.

Anti-GMP 140 antibody

The S12 antibody developed by McEver and Martin (1984) is of particular interest since it binds only to activated platelets. Both whole antibody and the Fab' fragment have been studied in primate models. Increased uptake of these preparations have been visualised in sites of deep vein thrombosis, dacron grafts and balloon arterial injury. This work is yet to be validated in man.

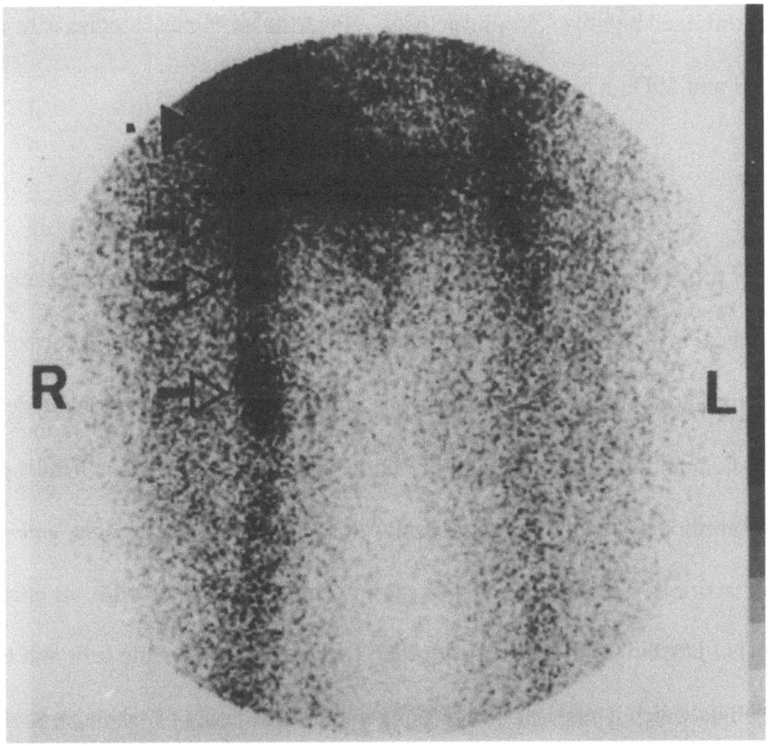

Figure 2. Anterior images of the thigh region of a patient following a balloon angioplasty. A band of increased uptake (open arrows) is visible showing platelet deposition along the mid portion of the right superficial femoral artery. Increased uptake is also visible at the haemostatic plug forming at the arterial puncture site (closed arrow).

Anti fibrin antibodies

Whereas antibodies reactive with platelets detect actively forming thrombi the use of antibodies associated with fibrin will localise and delineate both fresh and chronic thrombi. Several different antibodies of the IgG1 class have been raised against the amino terminus of the β chain of fibrin 11. Antibodies associated with fibrin are considered to have high specificity and high avidity however these agents are reported to have slow blood clearance and images have contained high background activity. Nevertheless clinical studies with antibodies such as T2G1s and 59D8 have been encouraging.

Discussion

The ease of preparation and radiolabelling of antibodies make their use especially attractive for routine clinical imaging investigations. The use of a monoclonal antibody for cell labelling represents a considerable advance over other currently available methods for the detection of abscess and inflammation and assessment of venous and arterial thrombi. Whilst the image quality using antibodies reactive with granulocytes would appear variable and the exact mechanism of action is not understood, this group of antibodies does offer an alternative to the use of In-111 labelling with the relatively high radiation dose to white cells and to Tc-99m HMPAO labelling which is restricted to imaging within four hours of administration. Further research trials will be necessary to evaluate which of the various radiopharmaceutical preparations is superior in clinical use.

The future use of antibodies for the detection of venous and arterial thrombi would appear especially promising. Clinical trials are still required to examine which of the relatively large number of antibodies is best suited for the detection of venous and arterial thrombi. In addition it will also be necessary to examine the effects of therapeutic agents such as heparin and thrombolytic drugs on the quality of the images. The Nottingham studies have generated considerable interest since the initial studies using the In-111-P256 Fab' antibody fragments in patients with peripheral arterial occlusion suggested that the images were capable of both localisation and characterisation of thrombi. The latter being of considerable value in patients referred for thrombolytic therapy. Since the success rate of thrombolytic therapy falls if the thrombus is not of recent origin a positive P256 image suggests suitability for thrombolysis.

One of the main limitations of the use of murine antibodies is undoubtedly the production of anti-mouse antibody responses, particularly since the patient population likely to benefit from these studies suffer benign (albeit life threatening) diseases. The reported results of clinical trials generally suggest that the production of patients responses to these materials is low, especially if antibody fragments is used. It would already appear that the advantages gained by the use of these antibody based radiopharmaceuticals outweighs any possible limitations. The use of these agents is likely to become widespread, revolutionising current radiopharmacy practice and heralding a new era in nuclear medicine.

Acknowledgements

We wish to thank our colleagues at University Hospital who participated in the Nottingham P256 studies, in particular Dr.M. Frier, Dr.M.L. Wastie and Mr. D Berridge.

References

1.Berridge DC et al [1989]. Local low dose intra-arterial thrombolytic therapy: the risk of stroke or major haemorrhage. British Journal of Surgery 76:1230-1233

2.Coller BS et al [1983]. A murine monoclonal antibody that completely blocks the binding of fibrinogen to platelets produces a thrombosthenic-like state in normal platelets and binds to glycoproteins 11b and /or 111a.Journal of Clinical Investigations 72:325-338 [1985]

3.Danpure HJ [1985]. Cell labelling with In-111 complexes.In Radiopharmacy and Radiopharmaceuticals Ed.A.E.Theobald. Taylor and Francis,London p.51-85

4.Frier M et al [1989]. Characterisation and clinical use of P256 Fab' platelet specific monoclonal antibody in the detection of arterial thrombosis. In Nuclear Medicine Quantitative Analysis in Imaging and Function. Eds.H.A.E.Schmidt and J.Chambron, Schattauer, Stuttgart.pp288-290

5.Gold HK et al [1988]. Rapid and sustained coronary artery recanalisation with combined bolus injection of recombinant tissue-type plasminogen activator and monoclonal anti-platelet GP11b/111a antibody in a dog model. Circulation.77:670-677

6.Hawkes RJ et al [1978]. Indium-111-oxine to label human platelets. Lancet 2:483

7.Joseph K et al [1988]. In vivo labelling of granulocytes with Tc-99m-anti-NCA monoclonal antibodies for imaging inflammation. Eur.J.Nucl.Med.14:367-373.

8.Locher JT et al [1986]. Imaging of inflammatory and infectious lesions after injection of radioiodinated monoclonal anti-granulocyte antibodies. Nuclear Medicine Communications 7:659-670

9.McEver RP and Martin MN [1984]. A monoclonal antibody to a membrane glycoprotein binds only to activated platelets.Journal of Biological Chemistry 259:9799-9804

10.Oster ZH et al [1985]. Thrombus radioimmunoscintigraphy:An approach using monoclonal antiplatelet antibody.Proceedings of the National Academy of Sciences USA.82:3465-3468

11.Peters AM et al [1986]. Clinical experience with Tc-99m-hexamethylpropyleneamineoxime for labelling leucocytes and imaging inflammation. Lancet 2:946-949

12.Stuttle AWJ et al [1988a. Use of an anti-platelet monoclonal antibody F[ab']2 fragment for imaging thrombus. Nuclear Medicine Communications 9:647-655

13.Stuttle AWJ et al [1988b]. In vitro studies with an anti-platelet antibody; P256. Nuclear Medicine Communications.9:813-815

14.Stuttle AW et al [1989]. Sequential imaging of post operative thrombus using the In-111-labelled platelet specific monoclonal antibody P256. British Journal of Radiology 62:963-969

15.Thakur ML et al [1988]. Monoclonal antibodies as agents for selective radiolabelling of human neutrophils. Journal of Nuclear Medicine 29:1817-1825

THE ROLE OF NUCLEAR MEDICINE IN THE EVALUATION OF THE PATIENT WITH ACQUIRED IMMUNE DEFICIENCY SYNDROME (AIDS)

Mrinal Mali and Leonard M. Freeman

Abstract

The Acquired Immuno - deficiency Syndrome (AIDS) was first recognized in the spring of 1981 in New York and California by the centers for Disease Control (CDC) (23). Subsequently there have been numerous invasive and non - invasive methods proposed for the early diagnosis and treatment of this usually fatal disorder. This article reviews the ongoing role of Nuclear Medicine in the diagnosis of HIV infection and HIV related diseases over the last decade as well as some recently introduced radionuclide investigations that are still in the realm of "work in progress".

Introduction

It was in 1981 that Gottlieb, Schroff & Shankar first described the Acquired Immuno - deficiency Syndrome (AIDS) in five young homosexual men. Since then there have been an increasing number of cases associated with high morbidity and mortality. Intravenous drug abusers and homosexuals have constituted the greatest risk groups. A June 1989 estimate from the Centers for disease control (CDC) indicates that there were 33,682 AIDS cases in the USA and the projection is that there may be as many as 270,000 AIDS cases by 1991. Longer range projections warn of a possible infected population of 1 - 1.5 million person in the USA and about 10 million world wide (21).

Etiology

AIDS is caused by HTLV III Human T - cell Lymphotrophicvirus or RNA virus classified into retrovirus group. It multiplies by RNA dependent reverse transcriptase into DNA in a limited number of cell types including lymphocytes, macrophages and cells of the nervous system. HTLV -IV or Simian T cell Lymphotrophic virus has been known to be a causative

R. P. Baum et al. (eds.), Clinical Use of Antibodies, 121–144.

agent of AIDS in Africa. One general classification that has been offered is as follows (21).

HTLV I & II cause of leukemia

HTLV III or HIV I or LAV (Lymphadenopathyassociated virus)

HTLV IV or STLV III (Simian T cell Lymphotrophicvirus) found in Africa. (Human T - cell Lymphotropic Virus -HTLV).

Clinical definitions and classification

An early observationwas that patients with AIDS had a specific impairment in the cell - mediated componentof the immune system and that they developed diseases predictive of this impairment. Recently laboratory and epidemiological evidence demonstrated retrovirus as a cause of immuno - deficiency with reversal of the T4/T8 ratio. Antibodies to the HIV virus was long demonstratedbefore clinical evidence of the disease. This led to a revision of the old definition of AIDS as a reliable diagnosed disease at least moderately predictive of underlying cellular immune - deficiency occurring in a person with no known underlying cause of reduced resistance associated with that disease. Revision of the AIDS definition resulted in a re-classification in 1987 that is now adopted world wide (24). It includes HIV encephalopathy previously called AIDS dementia complex ie Myelopathy and neuropathy.

HIV IN HEALTH CARE WORKERS (22,1).

Although HIV is not transmitted through casual contact, the potential for transmission always exists in health care workers, such as laboratory personnel, physicians and nurses. There has been a steady increase in health care worker exposure in spite of careful precautions. They include such things as an accidental needle stick, intimate contact with patient fluid or serum or exposure during surgery. To date there have been 1449 health care workers exposed to AIDS, with nurses being the group at greatest risk. The great majority of nurse exposures have been accidental needle injuries (80%) in patients rooms or clinics (64%). Risk of HIV sero conversion following needle stick is approximately 0.45% (2,22). Although this small number should provide some degree of comfort, continued diligence with all precautions should be practiced when dealing with patients or body fluids from patients with HIV infection.

TABLE 1

CDC CLASSIFICATION OF HIV INFECTION

Group I	Acute infection, Glandular fever
Group II	Asymptomatic HIV infection
Group III	Persistent Generalised Lymphadenopathy
Group IV	**Sub group A** Constitutional Symptom (fever, wt loss, diarrhea for > 1 month, formerly called AIDS related complex or ARC).
	Sub group B Neurological disease, HIV encephalopathy previously called AIDS dementia complex. (Myelopathy & Neuropathy)
	Sub group C Secondary infectious disease Pneumocystis carinii pneumonia Mycobacteria avium-intracellular (MAI) Oesophageal Candidiasis
	Sub group D Secondary neoplasm, Kaposi's sarcoma, Non Hodgkin's lymphoma Primary cerebral lymphoma.
	Sub group E Other conditions ie. clinical findings not classified.

Opportunistic disease

Patients with the acquired immuno deficiency syndrome (AIDS) present with a variety of infections. Almost any organism can become a pathogen in a person whose immune system has been devastated by the HIV virus. Protozoal infections are perhaps the most common of the opportunistic infections seen in patients with AIDS. In approximately 60% of AIDS patients, the initial diagnosis of AIDS is made following the discovery of Pneumocystis carinii (PCP) infection. The chance of having a single episode of PCP during the course of illness in an AIDS patient is 65% with a 10% mortality occurring during the first episode. Cryptosporidiosis is another protozoal infection that commonly affects the GI system and presents with severe watery diarrhea. Toxoplasmosis G is the next most common protozoan and generally presents with Encephalitis and/or brain abscess with multiple focal neurological deficits (34).

Bacterial infections occur less frequently in adults. The bacteria associated with a T cell defect are Listeria monocytogenes,salmonella and typical and atypical Mycobacteria.Infection more typically related to a B cell defect include streptococcus pneumonia and Hemophilus influenza.

Viral and fungal infections have variable presentations. Viral infections e.g cytomegalic inclusion virus (CMV) and Herpes produce high mortality and morbidity in comparison to fungal infection. Candida albicans, Cryptococcus neoformans, Histoplasma capsulatum are the commonest opportunistic fungal infections (34).

In pediatric AIDS patients, bacterial infections are a much more frequent cause of morbidity and mortality. Lymphoid interstitial Pneumonitis is currently recognised as one of the most frequent pediatric pulmonary manifestationof AIDS with Kaposi's Sarcoma being a much less common finding (4,14,15).

Kaposis Sarcoma (KS) is a multifocal systemic neoplasm manifested primarily by multiple vascular nodules in the skin and other organs. ExtracutaneousKaposi's Sarcoma (KS) involving the skin has a fairly rapid disease course resulting in death within two or three years of diagnosis. In contrast, classical Kaposi's Sarcoma has a rather more indolent course and remains localised to the skin. Kaposis Sarcoma is the most common neoplasm in AIDS that occurs in homosexuals/bisexualsand is relatively rare in heterosexuals (35).

The next most common neoplasm in order of decreasing frequency are non-Hodgkin's Lymphoma, Hodgkin's Lymphoma and chronic Lymphocytic Leukemia.

HIV encephalopathy, previously known as AIDS dementia complex and HIV wasting Syndrome are increasingly being reported as a complication of HIV infection (45). The clinical presentation are neuropsychiatric syndromes, dementia and focal motor and sensory loss with hypercatabolic muscular wasting.

Role of nuclear medicine

Non-invasive, easy to perform radionuclide studies have contributed to the early diagnosis of opportunistic infections such as PCP and AIDS related dementia. The remainder of this paper will concentrate on specific examples of Nuclear Medicine's role.

Gallium 67 citrate scanning

Gallium 67 citrate scans have assumed an important role in clinical management of patient with AIDS; particularly in those patients who suffer from fever and/or respiratory symptoms.

It is a highly sensitive means of detecting pneumocystis carinii pneumonia which is the most common life threatening opportunistic infection in AIDS, and has also aided in the diagnosis of a variety of other pulmonary infections including typical and atypical mycobacteria, fungi, bacteria and viruses, and has thereby deferred the need for costly invasive procedures (36,37).

Gallium-67 is produced in the cylotron by the bombardment of a target enriched in zinc-68 and has a physical half life of 77.9 hour. Patients are intravenously injected with Gallium-67 between 3-6 mCi (for children the dose is reduced according to the body weight) and scanned approximately 48-72 hours after injection. Though findings may be seen on early scans at 24 hours, later scans generally are preferred. Spies el al (5,17) studied 21 AIDS patients demonstratingthat 24 hour scans can diagnose PCP with a high degree of accuracy and provide a practical alternative to the standard 72 hour scan.

Normally Gallium is distributed within the rib cage, spine, scapulae, liver, spleen and excreted in the bowl particularly in the ascending and transverse colon.

Diffuse uptake of radiogallium

PCP has a variable presentation on Gallium scan of the chest, ranging from negative to total lung involvement and varying in intensity from minimally above background (1+) activity to greater than hepatic uptake (4+). Although there is much overlap in the Gallium scan presentation of PCP with other opportunistic infections, PCP is the most common lung infection detected. The most common abnormal pattern seen on Gallium scan in HIV positive patients is a diffuse homogenous uptake or activity (12,49). see Fig 1. Recently a different pattern of diffuse heterogenous Gallium accumulation in HIV positive patients with PCP was noted (13). Earlier Skarynski et al (26) had described this pattern of diffuse heterogenous lung uptake of Gallium with M.avium - intracellular infection. In Kramer et al's (13) study 77 Gallium chest scans showed diffuse uptake. Of these cases, 44% had diffuse heterogenous activity and 56% had homogenous activity. The diffuse heterogenous pattern had a high positive predictive value of 87% as compared to 64% when diffuse homogenous uptake was encountered.

Gallium scanning is superiour to chest radiographs in detecting PCP with a sensitivity up to 90% of overall cases and up to 86% in patients with normal chest X-ray (28). The specificity of Gallium scanning is low (52-54% overall), but maybe improved somewhat by using a grading system for intensity of pulmonary uptake (12,13).

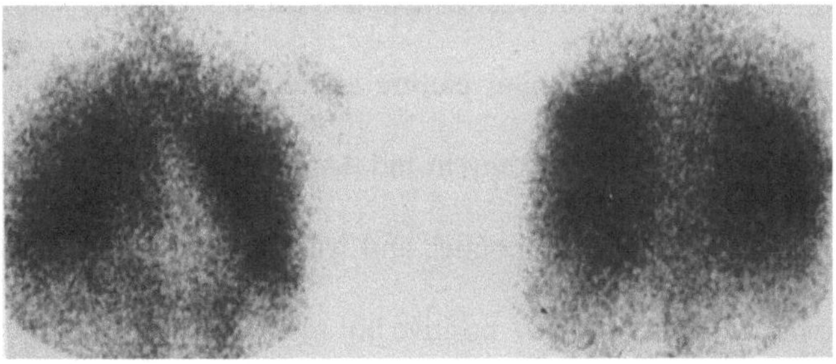

Figure.1 Pneumocystis Carinii Pneumonia - Diffuse pattern - anterior (left) and posterior (right).Gallium-67 citrate chest images show a 4+ diffuse uptake pattern.

Tuazon et al (20) used Gallium-67 scintigraphy to evaluate 20 patients with AIDS and suspected PCP. Lung uptake of Gallium-67 was demonstrated in 100% of AIDS patients with PCP including those with subclinical infections.

Barron et al (28) also evaluated the validity and reliability of Gallium scanning in diagnosing PCP in a study of 34 patients thought to have pulmonary complications of AIDS. The overall sensitivity for PCP detection was 94%, with a specificity of 74%. Among patients whose chest radiographs were normal or equivocal at the time of admission the sensitivity was 86% and the specificity was 85%. Based on a 49% prevalence of PCP in AIDS patients, positive and negative predictive values were calculated to be 77% and 93% respectively. Similar values were recorded for patients with normal or equivocal chest radiograph. It was concluded that a negative Gallium scan would indicate that there is only a 7% chance PCP is present. On the other hand a patient with a positive scan has a 23% probability of having an infection other than PCP. As elucidated by several authors, including Kramer(13), the diffuse pattern of uptake is also seen with Cryptococcus and Cytomegalovirus infection. In addition bacterial pneumonia or Tuberculosis may also produce a similar picture as non-infectious chronic inflammatory process like Sarcoidodis, drug toxicity (Bleomycin and Amiodarone), Radiotherapy, Pulmonary vasculitis, Pneumoconiosis, Uremic pneumonitis, and lymphangitic carcinomatosis. It is also known that cigarette smokers who are HIV positive but asymptomatic show diffuse uptake on Gallium scan (37).

In children, Lymphocytic interstitial Pnemonitis (LIP) currently is recognised as a frequent pediatric manifestation of AIDS (4,14,15). On Gallium-67 scan a diffuse pattern throughout the lung is indistinguishable scintigraphically from that of PCP. LIP would be one primary suspicion if this pattern is encountered in an HIV positive child.

As indicated earlier, the sensitivity and specificity of a Gallium lung scan for the detection of PCP is most often based upon zero to 4+ or 5+ grading systems (Table II). This is based upon the relative intensity of pulmonary uptake as compared to Hepatic uptake (13,19).

Coleman et al (25) suggested that increased intensity of uptake increased the specificity of Gallium scanning for PCP. Kramer et al (12,13) showed that the positive predictive value for PCP of a scan increased as the intensity of the pulmonary uptake increased from 64% (if all scans graded 2+ or higher were included as positive) to 77% (if only scans graded 4+ were positive).

TABLE 2

Grade I	Lung activity less than or equal to adjacent soft tissue
Grade II	Lung activity greater than adjacent soft tissue but less than liver
Grade III	Lung activity equal to liver
Grade IV	Lung activity greater than liver

Similarly the specificity increased only from 79% to 95%. In addition the frequency of higher intensity uptake was significantly greater when PCP was diagnosed than when other pathology was found.

Focal pulmonary and lymph node activity

Focal Pulmonary uptake of Gallium is a non-specific finding due to a focal inflammatory process as seen in bacterial pneumonia, atypical mycobacteria avium intracellular, mycobacterium Tuberculosis, Lymphoma and rarely in PCP (13,26,27). see Fig 2.

Focal Lymph node activity is a common abnormality seen on Gallium scans. Most frequently seen are hilar, mediastinal and para-aortic nodes (9,46). Focal lymph node uptake is not specific for any particular disease process, but it occurs in infection with M.Tuberculosis, M.Avium intracellular, and CMV as well as in superimposed neoplasm such as Hodgkin's disease and Lymphoma (9,13). see Fig.3.

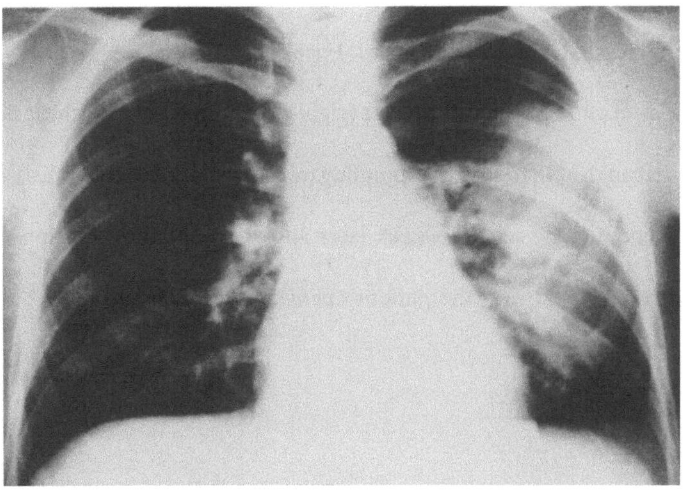

Figure 2a Pneumocystis Carinii Pneumonia - Focal. Chest radiograph reveals a large, but relatively focal, infiltrate in the left mid-lung field.

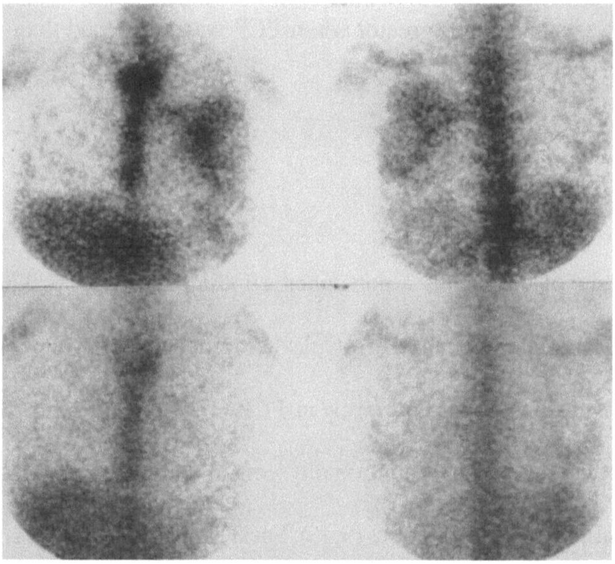

Figure 2b.Pneumocystis Carinii Pneumonia - Focal pattern

Upper row - Anterior (Left) and posterior (right) Gallium-67 citrate chest image show focal uptake in the left mid-lung field corresponding to the radiographic filtrate

Lower row - Repeat study several weeks later shows complete resolution of the abnormal activity.This correlated well with the patient's clinical improvement.

A variable pattern of focal uptake in atypical segments is now being reported in patients receiving aerosolised pentamidine therapy (38,39). Normally alveolar ventilation gradually increase from upper to lower lobes with blood flow increasing much more rapidly from upper to lower lobes (because of hydrostatic pressure). As a result the aerosolised pentamidine does not reach the atypical segments in a sufficiently high concentration and this permits the pneumocystis carinii to relapse in this region.

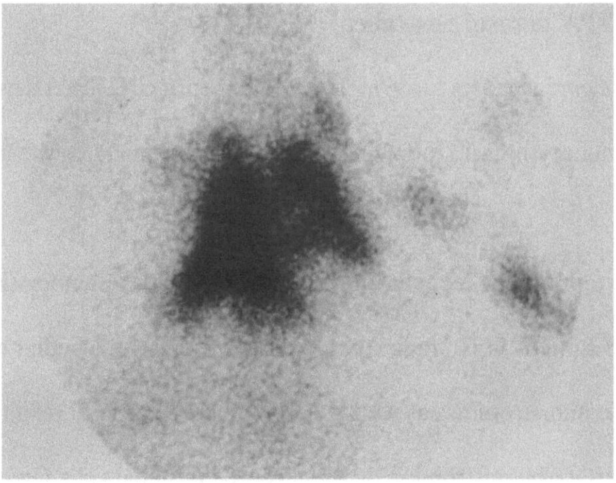

Figure 3. Hodgkins Disease Adenopathy in AIDS Patients Gallium-69 citate chest scan demonstrates several large areas of bilaterally increased uptake in the hilar, parahilar and left axillary region. Hodgkins disease was confirmed on biopsy

Negative gallium scan

A negative Gallium scan with a negative chest x-ray has a high negative predictive value for intrathoracic pathology. The negative predictive value for PCP with a negative Gallium chest scan is 96%. This combination of findings in a symptomatic AIDS patient should direct the search for infection away from the chest and obviate the need for invasive tests (9,13). A negative Gallium scan with a positive chest radiograph often indicates Kaposi's Sarcoma. The inability of Gallium to localise in areas of active Kaposi's infection has been observed by several investigators, including Kramer and Maddeddu (13,30). There is no specific explanation for this interesting observation.

Technetium 99M DTPA aerosol clearance

Increased thoracic clearance rates for 99m-Tc labelled pentate (DTPA) have been reported for a variety of inflammatory diseases following toxic exposures, including the long term effects of smoking (47).

Evidence was first reported by Yoneda and Walzer (18) that Pneumocystis pneumonias in rats accelerate the diffusion of horse radish peroxidase through the alveolar capillary barrier. This observation led to human studies as well (8,16). The onset of PCP results in a change in alveolar-epithelial interface by destruction of the Type I epithelial cells (Pneumocytes), with a resultant increase in lung permeability and subsequent replacement by Type II epithelial cells.

In a study from Doherty et al (6.7), lung permeability was measured using the mean transfer time (T50+/- Standard Error of Mean:"SEM")of nebulised 99m-Tc DTPA from alveoli to blood. The study group consisted of 126 asymptomatic HIV antibody positive patients (80 smokers, 46 non smokers), 30 HIV antibody positive patients with PCP and 20 patients (7 HIV antibody positive, 13 HIV negative) with an assortment of infection (10 mycobacterial, 5 streptococcal, 3 legionella, 1 staphycoccal and 1 unidentified infection that responded to erythromycin). 99m-Tc DTPA was inhaled in aerosol form in supine subjects, delivered by a Venticis II nebulizer (produces aerosol droplets that have mass median aerodynamic diameter of 0.9 um and geometric standard deviation of 1.5). Each lung was divided into thirds, (upper, middle and lower regions). Each region was corrected for its own background and 99m-Tc decay.

Transverse curves were initially analysed by applying a computer derived single exponential least squares fit to data. The mean transfer time (T50 +/- SEM) for patients with PCP (including smokers) was 2.1 +/- 0.2 min and for legionella was 3.2 min. In PCP effective treatment causes the transfer to slow (mean T50 changed from 22.7 +/- to 3.3 min) and became monoexponential. A very rapid transfer time with a biphasic curve indicated severe alveolar damage with a high probability of PCP and legionella (2 cases). The lung 99m-Tc DTPA transfer curve for bacterial pneumonia (other than legionella) had a monoexponential curve and were indistinguishable from those seen in cigarette smokers.

In a study from France (Picard and Associates) (16) results of 99m-Tc DTPA aerosol clearances were calculated in 11 AIDS patients suspected of PCP and were compared with those of Broncho-alveolarlavage (BAL). A submicronicmonodisperseaerosol (0.5 micron mass median diameter) of 99m-Tc DTPA (30mCi in nebulizes) was inhaled in the upright position over a 5 minute period. Sequential (1 min images for 20 mins) images in a posterior view were obtained with a Gamma camera linked to a computer.

For each lung, time activity curves were drawn and fitted with a monoexponential time using regression analysis for the first 7 min of the study. The pulmonary 99m-Tc DTPA clearance was calculated slightly differently from the Doherty study (6,7) and was expressed in terms of percentage decrease of radioactivity per min (% min-1). A clearance value was considered increased if it was higher than two standard deviations from the mean value in a normal non smoking subject (1.1 =/- 0.34% min-1, n=10). Nine patients with PCP had increased clearance five times higher than normal (5.6 =/- 2.3% min-1 vs normal). Only six patients had abnormal Gallium scans, while three others had normal or equivocal scans. One month after completing specific therapy three of four patients with PCP, had clearances that reverted towards the normal. However in one patient the clearance remained increased and lavage fluid analysis demonstrated persistent PCP.(In all four patients Gallium was normal).

The results of these two studies and various other studies clearly explains that 99m-Tc DTPA studies also are a sensitive marker of alveolar epithelial damage indicative of infection. Using the GAllium and/or 99m-Tc DTPA aerosol study, PCP in AIDS patients can be detected early and treatment instituted despite normal chest x-rays and arterial blood gases. Based on this, one can then decide to proceed with tests such as BAL, and hence prevent untoward complications of more invasive procedures.

Unfortunately the technique lacks some specificity, as increased lung permeability can also be seen in interstitial lung diseases, the adult respiratory distress syndrome, and legionella Pneumonia.

Advantages of the 99m-Tc DTPA aerosol study are that it is simple to perform even in severely ill hypoxemic patients, is rapidly analysed, tracer is easily available and it is a simple less expensive exam than other more invasive tests. It has a slightly greater sensitivity and specificity than Gallium as shown by Picard et al (16) and Kohn et al (36). It is easier to monitor a patients response to therapy and identify patients with a relapse.

99m-Tc human serum albumin intravenous studies

In a study by Brandhorst (48) 99m-Tc Human serum (HSA) albumin in millimicrospheres was injected intravenously and its uptake by macrophages in the lung was studied by scanning. In AIDS patients opportunistic lung infections have high macrophage concentration associated with epithelial damage. When HSA as millimicrosphere is injected intravenously it easily crosses the damaged alveolar-capillary epithelium into the alveoli and is subsequently taken up by macrophages within the lung. Normally this phenomena is not visualised due to the intact alveolar epithelial barrier.

Scintigraphy with 99m-Tc human serum albumin millimicrospheres are still under clinical evaluation. Images obtained 40 min after injection of Tc HSA and 3 days after Gallium injection were compared. Both scans were positive in 4 patients with confirmed PCP, both were negative in the three without lung infection; and neither scan was positive in 5 patients without PCP but with other lung problems. The 99m-Tc albumin scan was positive and Gallium was negative in one patient with diffuse malignant lymphoma of the lungs. Two patients who failed to receive Gallium scans (1 with varicella Pneumonia and 1 with mycobacteriosis)also showed positive 99m-Tc albumin scans. " It's quicker and you can start your therapies much earlier" according to Brandhorst.

Gastrointestinal activity

Gastrointestinal disease is the second most common type of disorder observed in AIDS patients. Colitis manifests as diarrhea, has been demonstrated to occur as a result of enteritis, secondary to Cryptosporidium, Karposi's sarcoma and other intestinal parasites.

Karposi's sarcoma, Lymphoma, or Burkitt's Lymphoma, and oral or rectal squamous cell carcinoma are some of the neoplasms that may localise in the GI tract. During the first 24 hours Gallium is excreted through the kidney and bladder. The next 24 hours fecal route predominates, thus making the interpretation of normal versus abnormal uptake somewhat difficult. Alternatively scanning with prior bowel preparation has been recommended. Indium-III leukocyte imaging is sensitive and possibly superior to radiogallium for the specific purpose of diagnosing gastrointestinal disease (11).

Neuropsychiatric manifestations

Clinical manifestationsof central nervous system AIDS include cognitive defects, memory loss and psychomotor retardation, (Often with frank dementia). Hypercatabolic muscular wasting with limb weakness, tumour and ataxia may also develop. This is known as HIV Encephalopathy(previously known as AIDS-dementia complex) (24).

Infections with Cryptococcus Neoformans, Toxoplasmosis gondi and cytomegalovirus may also cause central system lesions (10,29). Additionally, cerebral involvement with AIDs related malignancies such as primary cerebral lymphoma may occur.

Neurological and psychiatric abnormalities develop as a result of direct infection of diffuse brain tissue, primarily involving white matter and subcortical nuclei, with lesser involvement seen in cortical grey matter.

Non-Invasive imaging techniques such as computed tomography (CT) Magnetic resonance (MRI, single photon emission computed tomography (SPECT) and Positron emission tomography (PET) have been the major investigative techniques used to study neurological involvement associated with AIDS. CT may not be sensitive enough to show the early white matter changes that occur in the HIV infection of the brain, MRI has been shown to be superior in this regard.

With the development of Lipophilic radiotracers, that are measures of cerebral blood flow as well as metabolism, SPECT & PET have come to the forefront as useful techniques for diagnosing early manifestations of HIV encephalopathy.

SPECT imaging

Iodine 123 iodoamphetamine (IMP) and Technetium-99m Hexamethylpropyleamineoxine

(HMPAO) are the primary radiotracersthat have been used to measure regional cerebral blood flow (rCBF) with SPECT. I-123 IMP remains stable for 15-40 mins. during which time initial scanning with SPECT is performed. It subsequently redistributes (because the lung acts as a reservoir, slowly releasing the tracer) and hence blood flow dependent distribution is lost. In comparison, HMPAO another lipophilic agent crosses the blood brain barrier and immediately breaks down into hydrophilic poplar compounds which cannot diffuse back across the blood brain barrier. Both of these radiopharmaceuticalshave proven to be useful in detecting HIV encephalopathy.

Ell et al (40) first demonstrated the ability of SPECT with 99m-Tc HMPAO to reveal abnormalities in rCBF in two patients with HIV encephalopathy. The first patient was a homosexual man, with increasing lethargy, memory impairment and tendency to fall to the left. Psychometryconfirmed severe dementia with learning and memory defects and marked apathy. CT scan showed enlarged lateral ventricles and subarachnoid space. SPECT showed an abnormal pattern of uptake with reduced rCBF in both temporo-parietal lobes and the right frontal lobe. A second case with early encephalopathy had minor atrophy on CT. SPECT revealed reduced uptake in periventricularwhite matter, and also in the left parieto-occipital region and both temporal lobes.

Pohl et al (41) studied 12 patients with HIV encephalopathyusing 123-I-IMP (and in 4 of these patients also performed 99m-Tc HMPAO exams). Eight patients had diffuse cerebral atrophy on CT scans, and in 4 patients MRI scans were performed: 2 of these revealed atrophy and/or leukoencephalopathy. SPECT scans were abnormal in all 12 patients showing multiple or focal defects in rCBF. In those patients with focal defects on SPECT, the defects corresponded to the focal signs or symptoms in all but 1 case. In comparative cases, the HMPAO studies appeared to be superior to those performed with IMP.

Yudd et al (5) compared 123I-IMP SPECT and CT in 25 patients with HIV encephalopathy and found the nuclear medicine techniques to be the more sensitive test. CT scans showed white matter hypodensities in one patient and diffuse atrophy in six, but appeared normal in 15 patients. The SPECT studies were abnormal in all 15 patients. In addition the more severely afflicted the patient was, the more abnormal the scan tended to be.

The clinical presentation of these patients showed primary neurological symptoms in 7, and 8 patients had a combination of findings, see Fig 4.

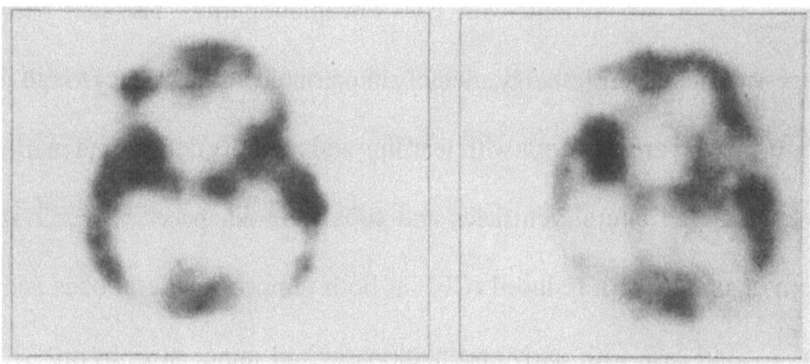

Figure 4. AIDS-related Encephalopathy

Diffuse patchiness and asymmetry is seen on the patient with AIDS (right panel). A transaxial SPECT image is shown. A comparable normal image is shown on the left (reproduced with permission from LaFrance NL et al: 1-123 IMP-SPECT in HIV-related dementia. Advances in functional neuro-imaging, MacMillan, Inc.)

PET scanning

As with any neurological disease i.e. Alzheimer's dementia and other acquired dementias, anatomical abnormalities occur later than functional changes. Hence it is during this stage of functional change that PET has been found useful to study altered perfusion of metabolism with the use of F-18 Fluoro-Deoxyglucose(18F-FDG).

Rottenberg et al (42) performed PET scans in 12 patients with HIV encephalopathy and 18 healthy control patients. Nine out of the 12 patients showed distinct patterns of abnormality. Early HIV encephalopathy was characterised by relative subcortical hypermetabolism. Progressive disease was accompanied by progressive cortical and subcortical hypometabolism.

Both techniques, SPECT and PET have shown early abnormalities not detected by CT/MRI and in this respect they are superior to these latter anatomic modes of imaging. Yet there is far more research and study to be done to establish the true sensitivity and specificity of these newer nuclear medicine modalities.

Radiolabelled human polyclonal and monoclonal studies

Experimental studies with a monoclonal antibody directed against the capsular antigens of Pseudomonas aeroginosa type 1, showed that specific immune imaging of microbial processes was possible (Rubin et al) (44). This observation led to studies with polyclonal human IgG.

In a study by Rubin et al, 128 patients with suspected focal sites of inflammation were studied. Intravenous Indium-111 labelled human non-specific polyclonal immunoglobulin (Sandoglobulin) was given. Indium-111 IgG localisation correlated with clinical findings in 51 patients with infection (21 with abdominal/pelvic infection, 11 with intravascular infection, 7 with pulmonary infection, and 12 with bone infection). In 63 patients clinically thought not to have infection, no focal localisation of 111-In IgG was seen. There were 5 false negative results and in 9 patients the data obtained were unusable. This study demonstratedthat 111-In labelled non-specific polyclonal IgG, if injected intravenously into patients with focal inflammation, accumulates sufficiently at these sites to be seen on scintigraphy. Human polyclonal IgG labelled with 99m-Tc as an alternative to 111-In labelling of IgG in febrile patients with AIDS has been used (3).

At present the use of 99m-Tc labelled antigranulocyte monoclonal antibodies to detect infection has attracted considerable interest (43). The technique does not require autologous labelling and appears to have high sensitivity and specificity. Yet this is still in its earlier stages and prospective comparative studies with more established Gallium-67 and Indium-111 WBC'S must be carried out.

At present, there is no available technique for detecting Kaposi's Sarcoma except for increased vascularity on angiograph or direct tissue sampling (35). Monoclonal antibody studies may prove to be useful in the area as well.

References

1. Lifson AR, Marcus R.[1988] Risk of HIV Infection for health care workers in the hospital. Medical aspects of Human Sexuality 1988 April 57-69.

2. Marcus R, and CDC Cooperative Needlestick Surveillance Group. [1988] "Surveillance of health care workers exposed to blood from patients infected with the human immunodeficiency virus". New England Journal of Medicine.319:1118-23.

3. Miller RF.[1990] 'Nuclear Medicine and AIDS'. Eur J Nucl Med.16:103-118.

4. Zuckier LS, Ongseng F, Goldfarb CR.[1988] "Lymphocytic interstitial pneumonitis". J Nuc Med.29:707-711.

5. Imaging News 'Nuclear Medicine refines therapy of Aids patients'. Diagnostic Imaging, Dec.1989;11-13.

6. O'Doherty MJ et al.[1985] 'Lung 99mTc DTPA transfer a method for background correction'. Nuc Med Commun.6:209-215.

7. O'Doherty MJ, Page CJ, Bradbeer CS.[1989] 'The place of lung 99mTc DTPA aerosol transfer in invg. of lung infections in HIV positive patients'. Respiratory Medicine 83:395-401.

8. Mason GR et al.[1987] 'Accelerated Solute clearance in Pneumocystis carinii Pneumonia'. Am Rev Respir Dis.135:864-868.

9. Bekerman C, Bitran J.[1988] 'Gallium-67 Scanning in the clinical evaluation of human immunodeficiency virus infection'. Sem in Nucl Med Vol XVII, No. 4.273-286.

10. Gilbertson V, Oates E.[1988] 'Gallium-67 imaging of unsuspected cerebral Toxoplasmosis in AIDS'. Clinical Nuclear Medicine Vol.13 No.9 Sept 1988.

11. Fineman DS et al.[1989] 'Detection of abnormalities in Febrile AIDS patients with In-III labeled Leukocytes and Ga-67 Scintigraphy'. Radiology.170:677-680.

12. Kramer EL, Sanger J. 'Gallium-67 scans of chest in patients with Acquired Immunodeficiency Syndrome'. J Nucl Med 1987;28:1107-1114.

13. Kramer EL. Sanger J.[1989] 'Diagnostic implications of Ga-67 chest scan patterns in human deficiency virus sero positive patients.' Radiology.170:671-676.

14. Sabbatani S et al.[1988] 'Ga-67 Citrate scanning x-ray computed Tomograph and chest x-ray in the study of interstitial pneumonia in patients with AIDS'. Nucl Med Commun.9:513-516.

15. Schiff RG, Kabat L, Kamani N.[1987] 'Gallium Scanning in Lymphoid Interstitial Pneumonitis of Children with AIDS.' J Nucl Med.28:1915-1919.

16. Picard C et al.[1987] 'Technetium-99m DTPA Aerosol and Gallium Scanning in Acquired Immune Deficiency Syndrome.' Clinical Nuclear Medicine July.12:501-5.

17. Spies WG. 'Gallium-67 citrate imaging in acquired immunodeficiency syndrome'. J Nucl Med Technol 17:23-28.

18. Yoneda K, Walzer PD.[1981] 'Experimental pneumocystis carinii pneumonia in the rat:mechanisms of alveolar injury'. Brit J Exp Patho.62:339.

19. Woolfenden JM, Carrasquillo JA, Larson SM.[1987] 'Acquired Immunodeficiency syndrome : Ga-67 citrate imaging'. Radiology 1987.383-387.

20. Tuazon CV, Delaney MD, Simon GL.[1985] 'Utility of Gallium-67 scintigraphy and bronchial washings in the diagnosis and treatment of Pneumocystis carinii pneumonia in patients with the acquired immuno deficiency syndrome'. Am Rev Resp Dis.132:1087-1092.

21. CDC:Human Immunodeficiency virus infection in the United Sates: MMWR Dec 18 1987/Vol 36/No s-6.

22. Update: 'Universal Precaution for Prevention of Transmission of Human Immunodeficiency Virus and other Pathogens in Health Care Setting'. MMWR, June 24, 1988 vol.37, No 24, 337-387, 387-388.

23. Gottlieb MS, Schroff R, Schauber HM.[1981] 'Pneumocystis carinii pneumonia and mucosal candiasis in previously healthy homosexual men'. Evidence of a new acquired cellular Immunodeficiency. N Engl J Med.305:1425-1431.

24. CDC: Revision of the case definition of acquired immune deficiency syndrome for national reporting: United States, MMWR 1985;34:373-375.

25. Coleman DL, Hattner RS, Luce JM.[1984] 'Correlation between Gallium lung scans and fiberoptic bronchoscopy in patients with suspected pneumocystis carinii pneumonia and the acquired immunodeficiency syndrome'. Am Rev Resp Dis.130:1166-1169.

26. Skarzynski JJ et al.[1987] 'Patchy uptake of Gallium in the lungs of AIDS patients with atypical mycobacteria infection'. Clin Nucl Med.12:507-509.

27. Mehta AL, Spies WG, Spies SM.[1987] 'Utility of Gallium scintigraphy in AIDS' (Abstract) Radiology.165:72-73.

28. Barron TF et al.[1985] 'Pneumocystis carinii pneumonia studied by Gallium-67 scanning'. Radiology.154:791-793.

29. Mc Lean RG, Murray IPC.[1984] 'Gallium scintigraphy in cerebral Toxoplasmosis'. Clin Nucl Med.10:592.

30. Maddeddu G et al.[1978] "Scintigraphic evaluation of Karposi's sarcoma'. Dermatologica 156:332-340.

31. Kotler et al.[1984] "Enteropathy associated with acquired immunodeficiency syndrome'. Ann Intern Med.101:421-428.

32. Castro MD, Ann MH, Curran JW.[1986] 'The Acquired Immunodeficiency Syndrome : Epidemiology and risk factors for transmission'. Med Clin of North America.70:635-649.

33. Murray JF et al.[1987] 'Pulmonary complications of the Acquired Immunodeficiency Syndrome : an update. Am Rev Resp Dis.135:504-509.

34. Kaplan LD, Wolfsy CB, Volberding PA.[1987] 'Treatment of patients with acquired immunodeficiency syndrome and associated manifestation. JAMA.257:1367-1374.

35. Krown SE.[1988]'AIDS associated Kaposi's sarcoma : pathogenesis, clinical course and treatment'. Editorial Review.AIDS 2:71-80.

36. Kohn H et al.[1989] 'Value of nuclear medicine procedures for diagnosis of opportunistic lung infections in AIDS patients'. Eur J Nucl Med.15:442.

37. Stafianakis GN et al.[1989] 'Increased Gallium-67 pulmonary activity in human immunodeficiency virus (HIV) positive non AIDS, non ARC, non-iv drug abusers : correlation with tobacco smoking'. J Nucl Med.29:829.

38. Bradburne RM et al.[1989] 'Relapse of Pneumocystis carinii pneumonia in the upper lobes during aerosol pentamidine prophylaxis'. Thorax.44:591-593.

39. McCandles BK, Cooper JA.[1989] 'Apical pattern of Ga-67 lung uptake in patients with acquired immunodeficiency syndrome treated with aerosolized pentamidine'. J Nucl Med 30:744.

40. Ell PJ, Costa DC, Harrison M.[1987] 'Imaging cerebral damage in HIV infection'. Lancet II.569-570.

41. Pohl P et al.[1988] 'Single photon emission computed tomography in AIDS dementia complex'. J Nucl Med.29:1382-1386.

42. Rotternberg DA et al.[1987] 'The metabolic pathology of AIDS dementia complex'. Ann Neural.22:700-706.

43. Kroiss A et al.[1989] 'Clinical application of Tc-99m labeled granulocytes antibody in bone and joint diseases'. Eur J Nucl Med.15:409.

44. Rubin RH, Young LS, Hansen WP.[1988] 'Specific and nonspecific imaging of localised Fisher immunotype 1. Psuedomonas aeroginosa infection with radiolabelled monoclonal antibody'. J Nucl Med 1988.651-656.

45. Navia BA, Jordan BO, Price RW.[1986] 'The AIDS dementia complex. I. Clinical features Ann Neurol.19:517-524.

46. McNeil BJ et al.[1981] 'A prospective study of computed tomography, ultrasound and gallium imaging in patients with fever'. Radiology.139:647-653.

47. Platner JW, Morrow PE.[1989] 'Altered clearance of inhaled 99m-Tc-Pentetate Aerosols following exposure to Cadmium Chloride Aerosols in Ferrets'. Exp Lung Res.15:77-91.

48. Brandhorst GH et al.[1988] 'AIDS and Nuclear Medicine (Experiences in Frankfurt and present status)'. Der Nuklearmediziner.Nr4,11:287-298.

49. Bitran J et al.[1987] 'Patterns of Gallium-67 scintigraphy in patients with acquired immunodeficiency syndrome and the AIDS related complex'. J Nucl Med.28:1103-1106.

DETECTION OF INFLAMMATION/INFECTION USING RADIOLABELLED ANTI-GRANULOCYTE ANTIBODIES: POSSIBILITIES AND LIMITATIONS

D.L.Munz, D.Sandrock, A.J. Morguet and A.Enderle

Various radiopharmaceuticals with more or less specific potential for detecting and localising inflammatory/infectious disease have been tested during the past decade or introduced recently (Table 1).

Since the introduction of I-123 (1) and Tc-99m (2) labelled monoclonal anti-NCA-95 (non specific cross reacting antigen)/CEA (carcinoembryonic antigen) antibodies for imaging inflammatory lesions, and more recently the use of the Tc-99m anti-NCA-95 CEA in bone marrow imaging (3,4) a relatively large number of investigators have reported on data obtained in patients with various benign and malignant diseases (5).

Both the I-123 antibody AK 47 (Granuloszint [r] Mallinckrodt Diagnostica, Hennef/Seig, Germany) and the Tc-99m antibody BW 250/183 (Scintimun [r] Granulozyt, Behringwerke AG, Marburg, Germany) are murine monoclonal IgG1 isotopes. For further details, see Table 2. NCA-95 represents a differentiation antigen of granulopoiesis and is expressed in cytosol and on plasmalemma starting with the promyelocytes. There is a 90:1 ratio between NCA-95-positive cells and neutrophilic granulocytes in human bone marrow. Immunohistological and fluorescence activated cell sorter studies revealed that promyelocytes took up only a very small amount of antibodies after intravenous administration of 1 mg Tc-99m BW 250/183. In contrast, myelocytes and more mature cells were targeted almost selectively at their cell membranes. The binding capacity was not saturated by the 1 mg dose (6). The high affinity, especially of BW 250/183 seems to explain the very rapid and stable antibody binding by bone marrow cells. Of the peripheral blood leucocytes, granulocytes can be labelled with an efficiency of about 96% as apposed to monocytes and lymphocytes which are labelled to less than 5% (7).

The vast majority of clinical data available up to now testing anti-granulocyteantibodies are related to inflammatory bone disease (without or following operative intervention). The

R. P. Baum et al. (eds.), Clinical Use of Antibodies, 145–150.

Table 1. Tracers for Inflammatory Disease.

Tc-99m MDP

GA-67 Citrate

Tc-99m Nanocolloid

In-111 Oxine [Tropolone, Acetylacetone] Granulocytes

Tc-99m HMPAO Granulocytes

Tc-99m Anti-granulocyte monoclonal antibody

I-123 Antigranulocyte monoclonal antibody

Tc-99m Polyclonal human immunoglobulin

In-111 Polyclonal human immunoglobulin

Agents for labelling: lymphocytes
Monocytes/macrophages
Bacteria [e.g. Staphylococcus Aureus]
Fungi [e.g. Candida Albicans]
Other micro organisms

Table 2. Characterisation of two different antigranulocyte antibodies.

	Monoclonal Antibody	
	Bw 250/183	AK 47
Subclass	IgG1	IgG1
Antigen	NCA-95	NCA-95
Binding sites/Granulocyte	7.1×10^5	7.1×10^5
Association constant[1/M]	2×10^9	3×10^8
Protein dose [μg]	100-400	120
Radionuclide	Tc-99m	I-123
Activity [MBq]	185-740	148-185

sensitivities and specificities range between 50 and 100% primarily depending on the location (limb vs spine) and floridity resp. age (acute, subacute or chronic) of the inflammatory process (5). The most important conclusions to be drawn from those studies are:

1) It is practically impossible to differentiate between septic and aseptic inflammatory disease.
2) Chronic inflammatory disease usually presents as cold lesion.
3) Inflammatory disease in spine usually presents as cold lesion. This is especially true for specific inflammation.
4) Normal activity distribution excludes inflammatory disease with a high degree of accuracy. In bones harbouring dematopoietically active bone marrow the inflammatory focus can often be detected and localised only by subtracting activity accumulated in uninvolved marrow or by kinetic analysis ending up in sensitivities and specificities 90-100% respectively (manuscript in preparation).

First reports available from prospective studies on patients with suspected subacute endocarditis, brain abscess subsequent to neurosurgical intervention and sinusitis point at sensitivities and specificities ranging between 80 and 100% each (manuscripts in preparation). There are no prospective studies reported on or published regarding the diagnostic usefulness of anti-granulocyte antibodies in detecting and localising occult abscesses as well as in assessing activity or extent of inflammatory lung and bowel disease.

In the following, we try to help clarify some of the mechanisms of targeting inflammatory foci by applying anti-granulocyte antibodies implying their diagnostic possibilities and limitations.

Assuming the total number of granulocytes in peripheral blood is 7.0 G/1 and the blood volume is 5 litres, the total number of granulocytes in a patient amounts to about 3.5 x 10^{10}. If each granulocyte expresses 10^5 epitopes, 3.5x 10^{15} epitopes can be labelled with the antibody. Injection of 0.2 - 1.0 mg of an intact antibody with a molecular weight of 150 kD translates to the injection of 0.8-4 x 10^{15} antibody molecules. Thus, the number of antibody molecules administered is of the same order of magnitude as the available epitopes. This circulation implies that particularly in patients with only slightly increased granulocyte levels, almost all of the circulating granulocytes can be labelled in vivo.

Escalating doses (0.25mg, 0.5mg. 1mg) of Tc-99m BW250/183) did not result in a change of peripheral granulocyte concentrations (8). I-123 AK 47 and Tc-99m BW 250/183 did not induce any complement activation or complement-mediated lysis. In vitro studies of phagocytosis and the killing of microorganisms, pinocytosis of colloidal gold, superoxide anion production, and lysosomal enzyme secretion have revealed that binding of both antibodies to the NCA-associated epitope does not impair or inhibit these granulocyte-specific functions (for details see 5). A sham dialysis model has demonstrated the viability of Tc-99m BW 250/183 labelled granulocytes in vivo (8).

The advantage of the Tc-99m or I-123 anti-NCA-95 antibodies are the lower radiation exposure (e.g the total body dose of Tc-99m BW 250/183 and I-123 AK 47 is about 0.0005 - 0.0015 mGy/MBq as compared to 6.168 mGy/MBq induced by In-111 OG: (7) and the simple handling without a necessary cell separation. Furthermore, the good physical characteristics of Tc-99m or I-123 and the overall availability of Tc-99m at low cost are of great advantage.

From a simultaneous intra individual comparative study on kinetics and biodistribution of in vitro In-111 oxine labelled granulocytes (OG) and in vivo Tc-99m anti-NCA-95 BW 250/183 labelled granulocytes (AGAb) performed by our group (9) we obtained insight into the concordant and discordant behaviour of those tracers. Compared to In-111 OG, Tc-99m AGAb demonstrated the following:

a) Faster activity clearance from peripheral blood
b) A smaller difference between cell bound and plasma activity (5-30% labelling efficiency in vivo)
c) Higher activity accumulation in bone marrow and soft tissue
d) Lower activity accumulation in kidneys and excretion in urine (about 20%/24 hours) and
f) A slower but more intense activity accumulation in florid inflammatory lesions in the lower limbs. The contrast of inflammatory foci however was worse in most cases due to the higher activity in the surrounding soft tissue.

Our analysis of the kinetics of Tc-99m AGAb BW 250/183 in bone marrow and inflammatory lesions in more detail led us to the conclusion that most of the in vivo labelled granulocytes take up the antibody in bone marrow (about 60-80% of NCA-95 positive cells are located in bone marrow), in the spleen (about 50% of the marginating granulocyte pool is located in the red pulp of the spleen), and possibility in the liver. The labelled granulocytes then leave these organs and migrate to a variable degree into florid inflammatory lesions. Thus, in spite of the theoretical possibility discussed above of labelling all circulating granulocytes (the circulating granulocytes pool represents about 50% of the total blood granulocyte pool) only a relatively small percentage of these cells is labelled in vivo while circulating.

In patients with inflammatory bone and bowel disease and in patients suffering from solid neoplasms and malignant systemic disorders, the maximum of activity in bone marrow (sacroiliac region as reference) was reached between 2 and 24 hours followed by a more or less rapid decrease reflecting emigration of labelled granulocytes (manuscript in preparation). These data open up a wide spectrum of kinetic studies on granulopoiesis and migration of granulocytes in various malignant and benign disease. An interrelationship exists between spleen and bone marrow in addition to the well-known relation between lungs and spleen. Very low or even absent splenic uptake could be observed in extensive septic disease and in a number of patients with AIDS (own observations: G Hor, personal communication). Hence, activity accumulation in the spleen following anti-NCA-95 antibody administration might be of diagnostic importance to assess the disease state in AIDS patients.

As mentioned above, after simultaneous administration of In-111 OG and Tc-99m AGAb, the latter demonstrated a slower but more intense activity accumulation in florid inflammatory foci in the lower limbs. These data indicate that there is some nonspecific exudation of Tc-99m AGAb into the inflammatory focus in addition to the immigration of granulocytes which have taken up their label primarily in bone marrow and spleen. These mechanisms are thought to be responsible for the localisation of florid granulocytic inflammatory foci.

In Crohn's disease or ulcerative colitis, a cross-reactive binding to CEA might take place, since CEA is elevated in these disorders not only in serum (in about 30% of patients) but also in bowel mucosa (7,8). As opposed to In-111 OG, there was no activity accumulation in the bowel lumen following Tc-99m AGAb (7). This result might be due to binding of the antibody to CEA in the bowel mucosa and/or formation of large antibody-granulocyte complexes in the bowel wall which are no longer able to enter the bowel lumen (7). Therefore, the significance of anti-NCA-95 monoclonal antibodies for the assessment of activity in Crohn's disease and ulcerative colitis is a matter of debate. The same is true for differentiating between abscesses and bowel inflammations and the detection of abscesses with internal communications (7).

It remains to be elucidated whether a certain degree of saturation of the NCA-95 epitopes on the granulocyte surface by the corresponding antibodies can impair or inhibit typical migratory functions such as homing to target tissues via specific receptors. Furthermore, the development of human anti-murine antibodies (HAMA) (5) must be kept in mind, in particular for follow-up studies, even though no immunologic or toxic adverse reactions have been observed after repetitive antibody administration (5,10). Promising developments in amaging inflammation are monoclonal antibodies against lymphocytes (whole population or their different subsets), mononuclear phagocytes and distinct microorganisms (Table 2) in order to make possible the noninvasive detection and localisation and/or assessment of activity and extent of different types of inflammation/infection. The significance of immuno-positron-emission-tomographyor immuno-magnetic-resonance-tomographyis at present only based on fiction.

References

1. Locher J.T. et al.[1985] Imaging of inflammatory and infectious lesions after injection of radioiodinated monoclonal antigranulocyte antibodies.Nucl.Med.Commun.7.659-670

2. Joseph K. et al.[1987]In-vivo-Markierung von Granulozyten mit Tc-99m-markierten monoklonalen Antikorpern: erste klinische Ergebnisse.Nuc.Compact18.223-226

3. Reske S.N. et al.[1989]Radioimmunoimagingfor diagnosis of bone marrow involvement in breast cancer and malignant lymphoma.Lancet I.299-301

4. Munz D.L. et al.[1990] Comparison of immunoscintigraphyand colloid scintigraphyof bone marrow.Lancet 336.258-259

5. Becker W. Wolf F.[1989].Immunszintigraphievon Blutzellen.Nucl Med.28.148-159

6. Reske S.N. et al.[1990] Verteilung von Tc-99m-markierten monoklonalen Anti-NCA-95/CEA-Antikorpern im normalen menschlichen Knochenmark.Nucl.Med.29.A23-A24 (Abstract)

7. Becker W.[1990].Immunoscintigraphyof infectious lesions. In: Munz D.L. Emrich D (Eds.) Immunoscintigraphy - Facts and Fiction. Excerpta Medica International Congress Series, Elsevier Science Publishers, Amsterdam - New York - Oxford.159-171

8. Becker W. et al.[1989] Kinetic data of invivo labelled granulocytesin humans with a murine Tc-99m labelled monoclonal antibody.Eur.J.Nucl.Med.15.361-366

9. Laue-Savic A. et al.[1989] Simultaneous comparison of biodistribution of 111-oxine granulocytes and 99m-Tc anti-granulocyte antibodies. In: Schmidt H.A.E., Buraggi G.L. (Eds.):NuclearMedicine,Suppl.25: Trends and Possibilities in Nuclear Medicine. Schattauer, Stuttgart - New York.110-113

10. Munz D.L. et al.[1990] Immunszintigraphie bei nicht-tumorosen Krakheitsbildern: Gegenwartiger Stand und Ausblick.Dtsch. Med.Wschr.115.147-153.

A NEW MARKER FOR THE DETECTION OF ADENOCARCINOMAS BY RADIOIMMUNOSCINTIGRAPHY

A.A. Noujaim, T.R. Sykes, A.J. McEwan, G.D. McClean, S.A. McQuarrie, G. Stanczyk and B.M. Longnecker

Introduction

Soon after the introduction of monoclonal antibodies (1) into the scientific domain, it became apparent that these probes has the potential to revolutionize the fields of immunoscintigraphy. The application of such technology in the field od oncology has recently been reviewed (2,3). Our interest in carbohydrate expression as tumour markers for adenocarcinomas (4-9) and squamous cell carcinomas was extended towards the development of a generation of monoclonal antibodies recognising unique markers. MAb 170, the subject of the present investigation, was derived after the immunisation of mice with the synthetic terminal disaccharide of asiaol GM_1. Clone selection was performed on human adenocarcinoma tissue sections. The exact nature of the natural epitope (CA 170) found on human tumours and which is recognised by MAb 170 is still under extensive investigation. The present study details the potential of this antibody as an imaging agent for a broad spectrum of adenocarcinomas.

Methods

a. MAb 170

The monoclonal antibody used in this investigation was provided to us by Biomira Inc. in either of two forms. The pure monoclonal MAB 170 was separated from ascites fluid which was certified as sterile, non-pyrogenic, mycoplasma and Mouse Antibody Production test (MAP) negative. The ascites fluid was purified by large scale ABx chromatography (J.T Baker Inc. Philipsburg, U.S.A.) and the material was then diafiltered into 67 mM Phosphate Buffered Saline (PBS) pH 7.2) buffer, diluted to approximately 2.1 mg/ml and sterile filtered prior to chelation as described previously (10). Radioimmunopharmaceutical MAb 170 kits were

R. P. Baum et al. (eds.), Clinical Use of Antibodies, 151–168.

radiolabelled with Tc-99m pertechnetate (~ 1.5 GBq) according to the manufacturer's instructions (Tru-Scint^{TM} AD, Biomira Inc., Edmonton, Canada). The chelated antibody was checked for immunoreactivity and the other biochemical parameters prior to use.

b. Immunopathology

We have tested a number of human tumour cell limes which can be grown in cell culture for their ability to bind MAb 170. Cells were obtained from the American Type Culture Collection (ATCC, Rockville, U.S.A.) and were readily cultured in standard medium containing RPMI 1640 with 10% fetal bovine serum and supplemented with L-glutamine, mercaptoethanol, and penicillin-streptomycin.

Cell seedings were usually done with 3-5 x 10^5 cells per flask which yield about 1-3 x 10^6 cells after one week under controlled incubator conditions at 37°C. At this time, the confluent adherent cells were harvested using trypsin-EDTA and assayed for viability (trypan blue exclusion), concentration, and total cell count. The freshly harvested cells were centrifuged, washed and resuspended in PBS at 2 x 10^6 cells per millilitre. A 100 μl aliquot was placed on a poly-L-lysine-coated slide and the drop allowed to air-dry. For immuno-cytopathology, a MAb 170 solution containing 10 μg/mL was then added to individual dry cell preparations and allowed to incubate for 15 minutes at room temperature. Each subsequent step was preceded by thorough washing in PBS to remove unreacted reagents. A second antibody (biotinylated horse antimouse IgG) was then added to the slides and incubated for a further 30 minutes to allow for reaction with antigen-bound MAB 170. The final steps consisted of the addition of horseradish peroxidase-conjugated avidin and the subsequent addition of the substrate (3'3 diaminobenzidine) to produce a large amount of insoluble dye at the original site of MAb 170 reaction with the tumour cell. The slides were then counterstained with hematoxylin, dehydrated, and mounted for interpretation. The slides were visually assessed as top the relative strength of staining intensity on a 0-4 scale as well as on the basis of percentage of total cells stained (0-100%) We have called the product of these two values the "Immunoreactivity Unit" (IRU) index.

For immunohistopathology studies, various tumour samples were collected at surgery and immediately frozen in a -70°C isopentane bath. The tissue was sectioned in a cryostat at -20°C to form 8 μm thick sections. The tissue sections were placed on poly-L-Lysine coated slides and used within 2 hours. The staining process was identical to that used for the immunocytopathologystudies.

c. BiodistributionStudies

Comparative tissue biodistribution studies were conducted using either Indium-111 or Tc-99m labelled MAb 170. For radiolabelling with In-111, and antibody solution in PBS buffer was reacted with DTPA cyclic anhydride with the resulting attachment of 1-2 chelate residues per antibody molecule. Unreacted and non-specifically attached residues were removed by purification on a G-50 mini-gel size-exclusion chromatographiccolumn. The preparation was lyophilized and kept frozen until further use. Radioindium attachment to the preparation was quantitative and resulted in a specific activity of 75-110 MBq/mg. Technetium-99m labelling of MAb 170 was accomplished according to the manufacturer's instructions (Tru-Scint^{TM} AD, Biomira Inc>, Edmonton, Canada) with radiochemical yields consistently greater than 90% as measured by thin-layer chromatography, and a specific activity of 0.75 GBq/mg.

Male Balb/c mice weighing approximately 20 grams were injected in the tail vein with MAb 170 solution containing 10 μg of antibody. Groups consisting of 4-6 animals were used for each experiment and the mice were euthanized six hours after injection. Selected organs were dissected from the carcass, blotted to remove adhering blood, weighed and then counted in a appropriately calibrated multi-sample gamma counter. Data was expressed as a percent of the injected radioactive dose per gram of tissue.

d. Clinical Trials

Preliminary clinical trials were conducted with ovarian (14) and colon (9) adenocarcinoma patients which were injected with up to 16 mg of wither In-111 or Tc-99m labelled MAb 170. Total amount of radioactivity injected was approximately 1.5 GBq for Tc-99m and 0.1 GBq for In-111. Cold antibody was admixed with the radiolabelled one to reach the desired antibody dose. The antibody was administered in 50 mL saline by slow i.v. infusion. Images were obtained at various time intervals post-injection and image reconstruction was conducted using a GE 400 AT tomographic camera. Whole blood samples were obtained from four patients recruited into the imaging trials with In-111 labelled MAb 170 for time periods up to 175 hours post injection and in the case of Tc-99m labelled MAb 170, blood samples were obtained from two patients for time periods of up to 24 hours. No separation of the labelled MAb from other blood proteins was attempted and all data was normalised to the injected dose. Data was analyzed using a non-linear least square regression program and a two-compartmentmodel was formed to adequately represent the elimination pattern of the radioactivityfrom the circulatory system.

Results and discussion

Natural Distribution of CA-170

The original selection of MAb 170 was based on its preferential binding to fresh frozen human adenocarcinomatissue sections using classical immunohistochemicalstraining methods. This approach utilises the natural tumour-associated antigen in native surroundings in a physiologically relevant matrix. Although the immunisation of the mice was effected using the synthetic asialo GM_1 terminal disaccharide (5), the final selection of the clone was determined by a combination of immobilized antigen as well as histopathology. A thorough study of the distribution of the antigen CA170 in normal and cancer tissues shows a highly restricted pattern with a primary expression on a subset of simple epithelial cells. In breast tumours, both ducts and acini epithelial cells showed moderate to strong immunoreactivity to MAb 170. While endocervical cells showed positivity, on the other hand exocervical cells were negative. A variety of cells of gastrointestinal origin (ie. colonic and gastric epithelium) as well as the collecting tubules of the kidney, liver bile ducts, and the epithelial cells of the lungs and prostrate also showed moderate expression of CA170. Pancreatic tissue showed reactivity in its exocrine cells and not its endocrine cells. The surface epithelial cells of the ovary demonstrated focal staining. Endometrial as well as sweat glands of the skin were found to express CA170.

A subset of simple epithelial cells including those of the proximal tubules of the kidney, hepatocytes of the liver, and alveolar cells of the lung were found to be unreactive to MAb 170. Stratified epithelial cells of the urinary bladder, skin epidermis, squamous epithelium of the esophagus, and epidermis of the exocervix were found to be devoid of CA170. However, the umbrella cells showed focal or luminal surface staining. Reactivity was not seen in the hematopoieticand germinal elements, in the neuroectodermalcells, including brain, spinal cord, melanocytes as well as the peripheral nerves. With the exception of a peculiar dotty staining of the smooth muscle cells of the uterine myometrium, the mesenchymal elements were found to be unreactive.

Human tumours showed a somewhat broader pattern of immunoreactivities particularly among tumours derived from simple epithelial cells. Thus, a strong expression of CA170 was noted in breast, colon, endometrial, lung, ovarian and prostatic carcinomas. Transitional cell carcinoma of the urinary bladder showed focal concentrations of CA170. Of interest is the observation that renal cell carcinomas were found to be unreactive since most renal cell carcinomas are reported to be derived from proximal tubular cells in the normal kidney. In this case, the normal kidney proximal tubules showed negative reactivity with MAb 170, All tumours of neuroectodermal origin such as astrocytomas and melanomas, as well as tumours of hematopoietic and mesenchymal origin did not express CA170. Table 1 gives the results of our histopathological studies on various normal and cancer tissues. Figure 1 is an example of a well differentiated adenocarcinoma of the colon showing malignant pseudoglands infiltrating the smooth muscle of the colonic wall. Figure 2 is that of a frozen section of a serous cystadenocarcinoma of ovary showing an intracellular pattern of staining. In general, one might conclude from this study that the pattern of immunoreactivity is that of cytoplasmic and luminal staining, with reactivities seen in secretions, indicating that the antigen may be shed. Preliminary biochemical investigations in our laboratory on the nature of CA170 indicates that the epitope recognised by MAb 170 on the natural antigen is associated with cytoskeletal proteins.

The scarcity of suitable fresh sections and their inherent heterogenicity imposes certain limitations in the quantitative study of the immunoreactivity of monoclonal antibodies. The selection of an appropriate human cancer line expressing the desired antigen becomes of important for two reasons: it allows us to identify a cell line source which would be subsequently used to develop animal tumour models in addition to the fact that such cell lines may very well present us with a natural source of the antigen for further characterisation. We have used in our study 18 cell lines from a variety of tumour sources. As can be seen in Table 2, there does not exist any correlation between the expression of CA170 in any one group of these lines and the corresponding distribution of the antigen as seen on histopathological specimens. This is not surprising since the metabolic requirements resulting in the surface expression of the tumour marker on the suspended cells are conceivably quite different from those which are necessary for the growth of the same cells *in vivo*. The use of immunoreactivity units (IRU) allows us a semi-quantitative method for the selection of the cell line with highest antigen expression. We routinely use the COLO 205 cells for standardising the immunoreactivity measurements of MAb 170 after chelation and radiolabelling. The same

TABLE 1

EXPRESSION OF CA170 IN NORMAL AND CANCER TISSUES

ORGAN	NON-CANCER			CANCER		
	TISSUE	# TESTED	# POSITIVE	TISSUE	# TESTED	# POSITIVE
G.I. Tract	Normal bowel mucosa	15	15	Colonic adenocarcinoma	53	53
	Inflammatory bowel disease	6	6	Colonic adenoma	6	6
	Small intestine (crypt)	3	3			
	Small intestine (luminal)	3	3	Gastric carcinoma	6	6
	Esophagus (squamous epithelia)	3	0			
	Esophagus (glands)	2	0	Stomach lymphoma	4	0
	Stomach-lumen	3	3			
Breast	Ductal epithelium	8	8	Breast carcinoma (ductal, lobular, medullary)	26	26
	Acini	3	3			
Ovaries, Cervix, and Uterus	Normal ovaries	8	2 *	Borderline malignancies	4	4
	ovarian cysts	8	7	Ovarian carcinoma	11	7
	Endocervix	5	5	Non-epithelial tumors	1	0
	Exocervix	4	0	Endometrial carcinoma	2	2
	Endometrium	4	4			
	Myometrium	3	0			
	Stromal cells	3	0			
Pancreas	Endocrine cells	3	0	Pancreatic carcinoma	1	0
	Exocrine cells	3	3			
	Ducts	3	3			
Prostate	Prostate	3	3	Prostatic carcinoma	1	0
Lung	Bronchial epithelial cells	6	6	Adenocarcinoma	3	3
	Alveolar cells	4	0	Squamous cell carcinoma	10	1
	Normal lung parenchyma	3	0	Small cell carcinoma	3	1
				Large cell carcinoma	1	0
				Adenosquamous Ca	3	1

EXPRESSION OF CA170 IN NORMAL AND CANCER TISSUES

ORGAN	NON-CANCER			CANCER		
	TISSUE	# TESTED	# POSITIVE	TISSUE	# TESTED	# POSITIVE
Liver, spleen	Hepatocytes	5	0	N/A	N/A	N/A
	Bile ducts	4	4			
	Kupffer cells	3	0			
	Spleen	3	0			
Heart	Myocardium	5	0	N/A	N/A	N/A
Adrenal	Cortex	3	0	N/A	N/A	N/A
	Medulla	1	0			
Kidney/ Bladder	Glomerules	3	0	Renal carcinoma	3	0
	Proximal tubules	3	0	Bladder carcinoma	4	1
	Collecting tubules	4	4			
	Bladder urothelium	3	3			
Skin	Epidermis	3	0	Squamous cell Ca.	2	0
	Adnexa	3	3	Melanoma	3	0
Nervous System	Spinal cord neuropil	3	0			
	Spinal cord neurons	3	0	Astrocytoma	2	0
	Brain Astrocytes	3	0			
	Brain neuropil	3	0			
Other	Tonsils	3	2			
	Skeletal muscle	3	0	Muscle sarcoma	3	0
	Lymph node	3	0			
	Bone marrow	3	0			
	Peripheral blood cells	3	0			
	Parathyroid	3	0			
	Anterior pituitary	3	3			
	Posterior pituitary	3	0			
	Thymus	3	0			

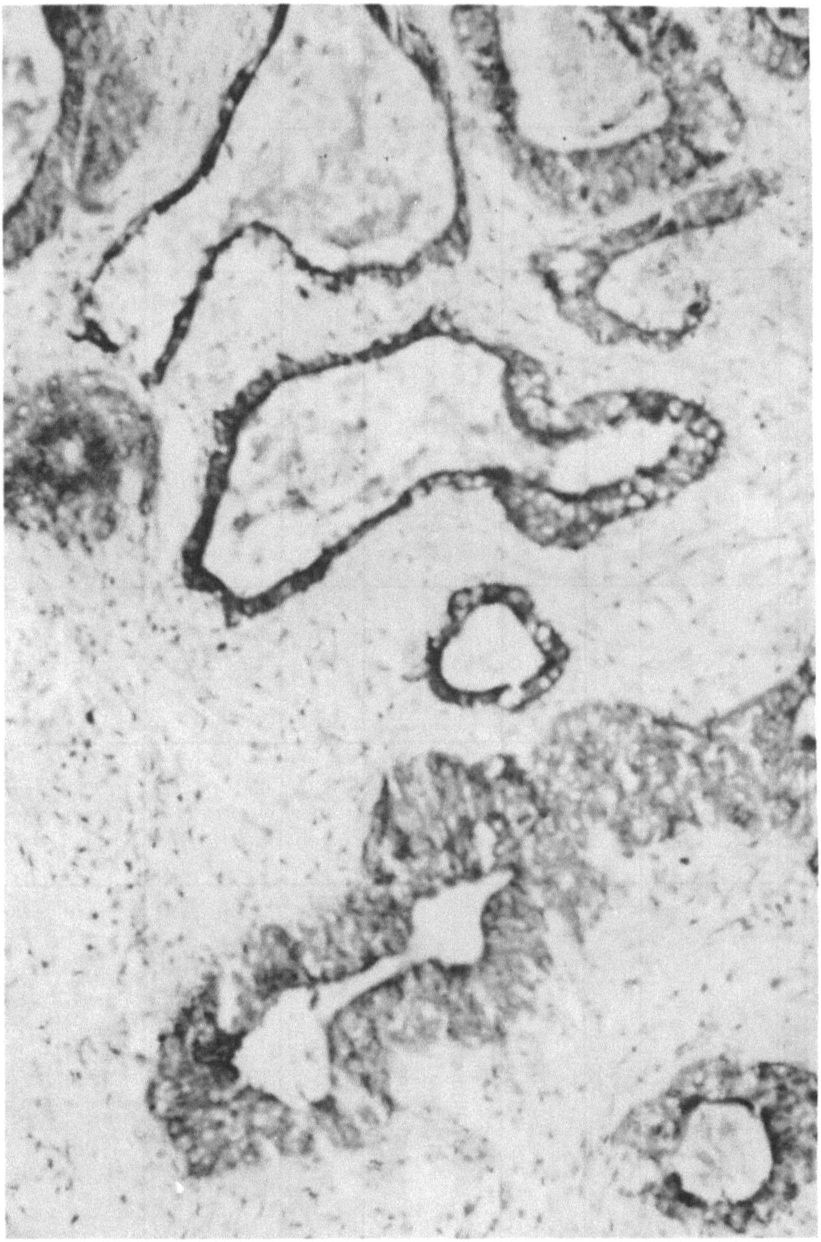

Figure 1. Adenocarcinoma of Colon - Frozen section after immunoperoxidase staining with Mab170

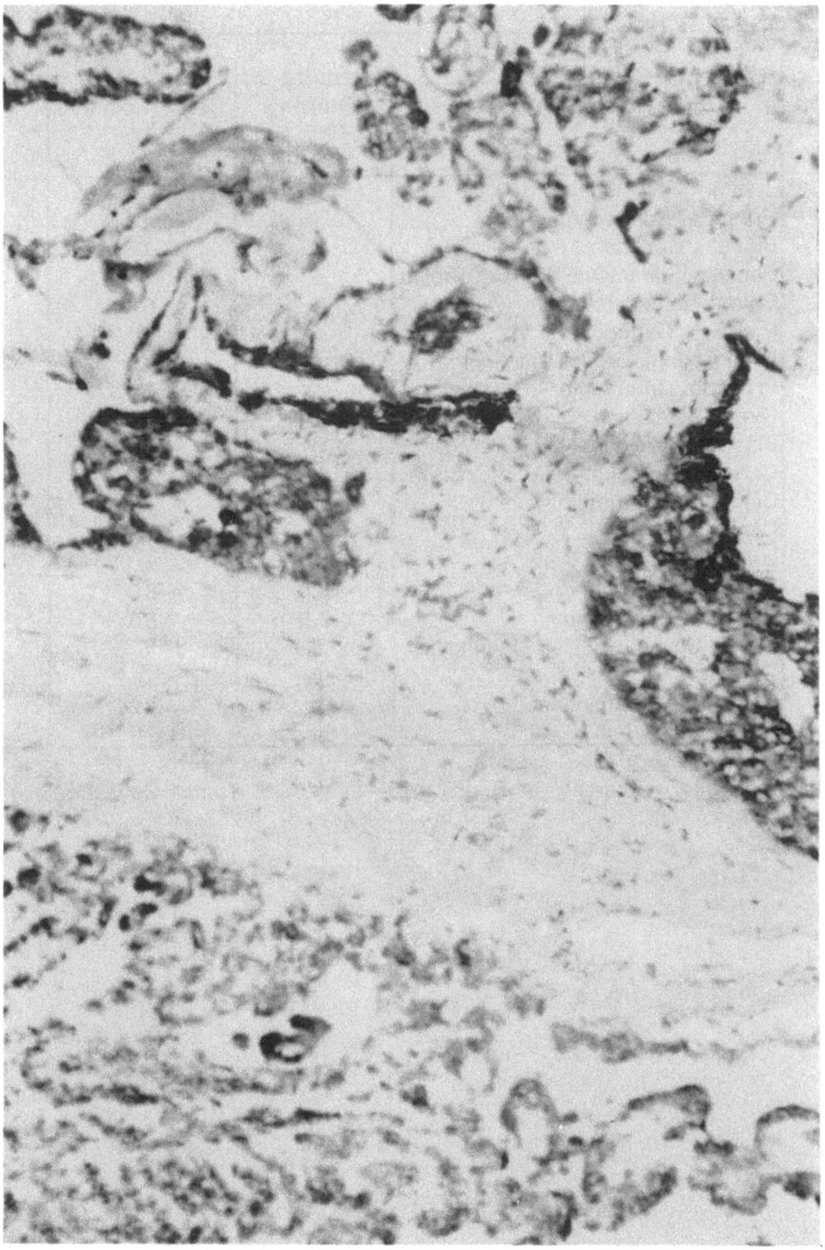

Figure 2. Serous Cystadenocarcinomaof the ovary - Frozen section after immunoperoxidase staining with Mab 170.

TABLE 2
IMMUNOCYTOCHEMICAL STAINING OF CULTURED HUMAN CELL LINES WITH MAb 170

Cell Line Designation	Tissue Type	Intensity of Staining	Percent of Cells Positive	Immunorea Units (IRU
LNCaP	Prostate Adenocarcinoma	0	0	0
SCaBER	Bladder Carcinoma	0	0	0
FaDu	Pharynx Squamous Cell Carcinoma	2	5	10
LS174T	Colon Adenocarcinoma	2	50	100
Du145	Prostate Carcinoma	0	0	0
SKMES	Lung Squamous Cell Carcinoma	0	0	0
PC-3	Prostate Carcinoma	2	50	100
CaOv3	Ovary Carcinoma	0	0	0
647V	Bladder Carcinoma	1	50	50
SIHA	Cervix Squamous Cell Carcinoma	0	0	0
C33A	Cervix Carcinoma	0	0	0
HT3	Cervix Carcinoma	0	0	0
SKLU1	Lung Carcinoma	0	0	0
MCF7	Breast Carcinoma	3.5	80	280
LOVO	Colon Adenocarcinoma	2.5	50	125
ME180	Cervix Squamous Cell Carcinoma	0	0	0
D54	Glioma	0	0	0
COLO205	Colon Adenocarcinoma	4	80	320

*Immunoreactivity Units = Intensity of Staining (0-4+) x % of Tumor Cells Positive (0-100%

TABLE 3

COMPARATIVE BIODISTRIBUTION OF RADIOLABELLED MAb-170 IN MICE*

TISSUE	In-111-MAb170	Tc-99m-MAb-170
Blood	24.3 ± 3.5	17.1 ± 2.3
Heart	8.1 ± 0.7	6.4 ± 0.9
Lungs	10.2 ± 0.9	6.9 ± 2.0
Liver	17.5 ± 3.7	9.6 ± 1.0
Spleens	7.2 ± 1.3	5.3 ± 2.5
Intestine	2.4 ± 0.6	4.0 ± 0.5
Stomach	1.3 ± 0.7	1.6 ± 0.5
Kidney	18.0 ± 2.4	14.0 ± 1.9
Bone	2.9 ± 0.2	2.7 ± 0.5
Muscle	1.0 ± 0.1	0.6 ± 0.1

* % injected dose/g, 6 hours after i.v. injection

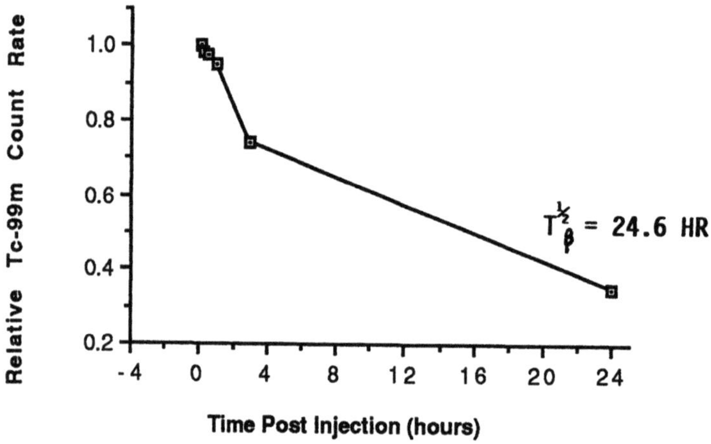

Figure 3. Relative Blood clearance of Tc-99m Mab170 in Humans.

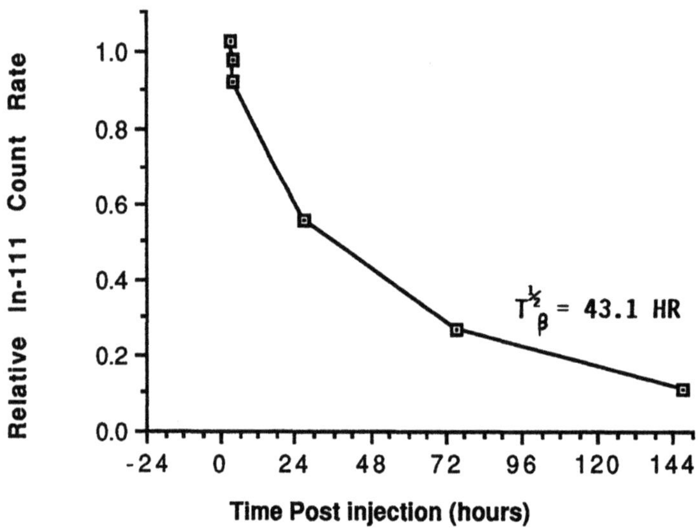

Figure 4. Relative Blood clearance of In-111 Mab-170 in Humans.

cell line is also presently used for the extraction and further characterisation of the natural antigen.

Biodistribution of MAb 170

A study of the bio distribution in mice (Table 3) of both Indium-111 and Tc-99m labelled MAb 170 reveals an interesting pattern comparable to our own observation where the same preparations were administered in humans. At six hours after intravenous administration, Tc-99m radioactivity levels in blood, heart, lungs, liver, spleen, kidney and muscle were lower than those observed in mice which were injected with In-111 labelled MAb 170. On the other hand, intestinal uptake levels of Tc-99m were significantly higher than those of In-111. Bone and stomach tissue levels of both tracers were similar. The above data can be explained on the account of the fast clearance observed after the administration of Tc-99m labelled antibody. Figures 3 and 4 of the pharmacokinetic assessment of blood levels in humans indicate both In-111 and Tc-99m clearance followed essentially a 2-compartment model while in mean terminal phase elimination half-life for In-111 was 43.1 ± 2.6 hours, that of Tc-99m was found to be 24.6 ± 0.5 hours. These levels were consistent with clinical observations of the blood clearance when patients were imaged sequentially. The considerable increase in liver uptake of In-111 by mice is not unusual given the tendency of In-111 to transchelate from DTPA chelates. The elevated intestinal uptake of Tc-99m may be partially explained on the basis that MAb 170 shows a tendency to bind to CA170 in normal colonic epithelial cells. This does not necessarily mean that *in vivo* accumulation of the same antibody can be expected after intravenous use. Of interest is that some biliary excretion of Tc-99m radioactivity has been noted in mice which were injected with Tc-99m MAb 170. We have not investigated if this radioactivity was associated with any biological fragment of the antibody in question and the assumption of active binding of the secreted radioactivity to the luminal surface of the intestines is speculative at best.

Clinical Results

Table 4 outlines the results from pilot imaging studies on 23 patients (14 with ovarian and fallopian tube adenocarcinomas, and 9 with colonic adenocarcinomas) to determine the potential utility of MAb 170 for detecting different types of adenocarcinomas and for the detection of metastases at different sites. While this particular study represents a very limited

TABLE 4

IMAGING RESULTS OF PATIENTS WITH OVARIAN AND COLON ADENOCARCINOMAS INJECTED WITH MAb 170

	OVARY / FALLOPIAN TUBE	COLON
No. of Patients (In-111)	8	5
No. of Patients (Tc-99m)	6	4
Total Sites Evaluated	79	45
True Positive	32	15
False Positive	0	1
True Negative	45	28
False Negative	2	1

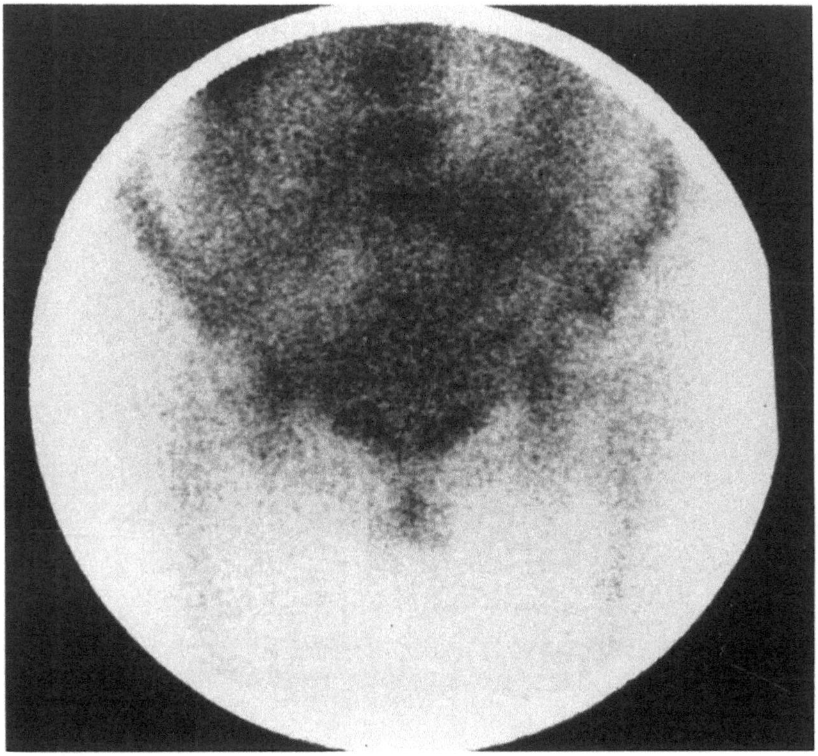

Figure 5. Primary Adenocarcinoma of the colon of a Patient injected with In-111 Mab 170

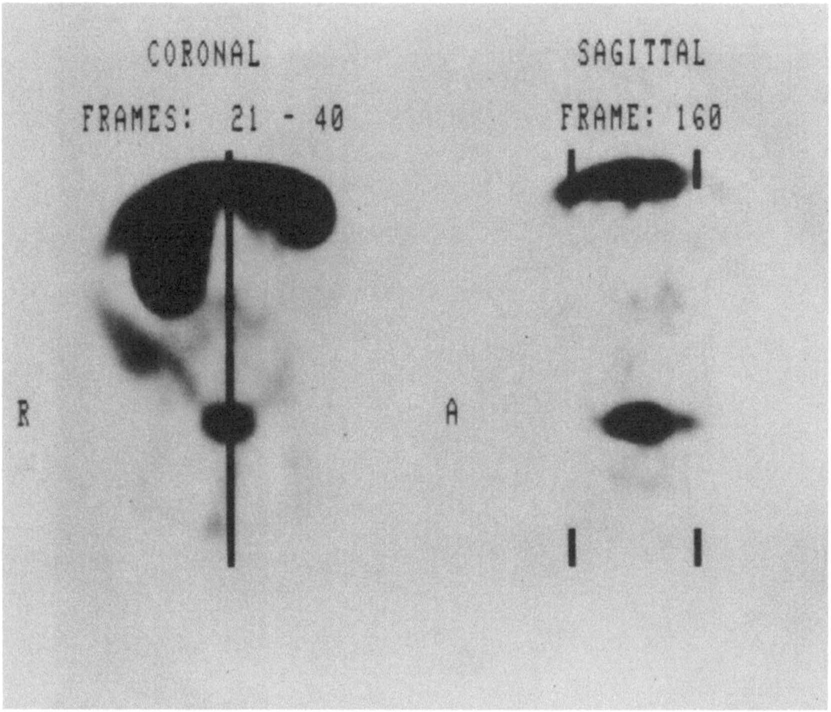

Figure 6. SPECT Scan of a Patient with metastatic ovarian adenocarcinoma injected with Tc-99m Mab 170

attempt to investigate the clinical utility of the antibody, the results have been encouraging enough to be the subject of much expanded clinical trials. In the present study, a total of 79 ovarian sites and 45 colonic sites of metastases were investigated. True positive images were defined as primary or metastatic lesions, defined by conventional radiological procedures, surgery or biopsy or by clinical examination which showed positive uptake of radiolabelled MAb. False positive images were defined as sites which showed positive uptake of the antibody which could be confirmed by any of the techniques described above, or on clinical follow-up over a three-month period. True negative images were defined on a regional basis. For example, if no disease could be demonstrated in the thorax by any of the techniques described above, and there was no evidence of antibody uptake, then this region was called true negative. Four regions were defined for each patient, thorax, abdomen, pelvis and other sites including bone and peripheral model groups. A false negative was defined as a primary or metastatic lesion defined by any of the techniques above described, which was not associated with positive MAb 170 uptake. Figure 5 is an example of a planar image of a patient injected with In-111 MAb 170 whereby a primary colon cancer shows a distinct uptake in the left iliac fossa consistent with a sigmoid primary. This was later confirmed at surgery. Figure 6 is a SPECT scan of a patient with metastatic ovarian cancer injected with Tc-99m MAb 170 at 22 hours post administration of the antibody. A coronal view reveals a residual mass posterior to the bladder. The sagittal section also shows a mass posterior to the bladder. This was confirmed by clinical examination and C.T.

Summary

The histopathological reactivity of MAb 170 with a broad variety of human adenocarcinomas as well as tumour localisation *in vivo* introduces this antibody as a useful pan-adenocarinoma marker probe. The technetium-99m labelled MAb, and its fast *in vivo* clearance allows for a rapid scintiscan for the detection of colonic and ovarian adenocarcinomas.

References

1. Kohler G. and Milstein C. Continuous cultures of fused cells secreting antibody of predefined specificity.[1975]. Nature (London) 256: 495.

2. Granowska M. Britton K.E., Radiolabelled monoclonal antibodies in oncology 1.principles. [1991].Nucl.Med.Commun.12: 65-76.

3. Granowska M. Britton K.E. Radiolabelled monoclonal antibodies in oncology 11. Clinical applications in diagnosis.[1991]. Nucl.Med.Commun. 12: 83-98.

4. Noujaim A.A. et al. A molecular approach to immunoscintigraphy:A study of the T-antigen confirmation in the surface of tumours. [1987]. Nuklearmedizin 26: 1-6 .

5. Noujain A.A. et al. Synthesis and experimental modulation of tumour-associatedantigens. New Tumour Markers and their MonoclonalAntibodies,[1987].R.Klapdor (ed) 8-16, Georg Thieme Verlag, Stuttgart, New York.

6. MacLean G.D. et al.A novel strategy to derive monoclonal antibodies for successfulimaging of cancer in humans. [1989] In: Cellular Basis of Immune Modulation. J.G.Kaplan and D.R.Green (eds) Alan R.Liss, New York, 587-599.

7. MacLean G.D. et al. The potential of synthetic tumour-associatedglycoconjugates(S-TAGs) for generating monoclonal antibodies for breast imaging and for specific immunotherapy,[1989]. In: Immunological Approaches to the Diagnosis and Therapy of Breast Cancer 11. R.L.Ceriani (ed) Plenum Publishing Corp. 3-11.

8. Samuel J. et al.Analysis of human tumour associated Thomsen-Friedenreichantigen.[1990]. Cancer Research 50: 4801-4808, August 1.

9. MacLean G.D. et al. Two novel monoclonal antibodies have potential for gynecologic cancer imaging. Antibody, Immuno Radiopharm (in press) 1990.

10 Sykes T.R. et al.Biological considerations in the evaluation of tumour-directed antibodies for radioimmunoscintigraphy.[1990]Proc.Symp on Radiopharmacol. D.J. Maddalena, G.M. Snowdon and G.R. Boniface (eds) 164-172.

NEW DEVELOPMENTS IN THE DIAGNOSIS OF AIDS AND STRATEGIES FOR THERAPY

G.V.Wangenheim and J.Lower

Acquired Immunodeficiency Syndrome (AIDS) is a new infectious disease which was first described in 1983. Since then, it has gained enormous attention in the medical community as well as in public, and it was probably the mostly discussed disease over the last decade. I therefore assume that the clinical symptoms and the time course are widely known.

for developing strategies for therapeutic intervention is the knowledge of the structure and the life cycle of the causative agent, the Human Immunodeficiency Virus (HIV). HIV belongs to the family of retroviridae whose genome consists of two identical single-stranded pieces of RNA each approximately 10kb in size. Those are contained in the viral capsid of which consists of numerous monomers of the viral main structural protein p24 (named according to its size of 24,000 D). A host cell membrane-derived envelope surrounds this capsid. A virus specific glycoprotein (gp-41) is embedded within this membrane, itself serves as an anchor for a larger outer envelope glycoprotein (gp120). In addition, the virus particles contain a few smaller structural proteins (p17, p15) whose role is not yet completely understood.

The life cycle of HIV is summarized in Table 1. Briefly, attachment of virus to the host cell is mediated by the viral outer envelope protein gp120 which recognises a cellular membrane protein as receptor. This cellular protein is known as CD4-antigen and is characteristic for the helper subset of T lymphocytes, although it is also expressed on the surface of a number of other cell types. In general, only these cells can be infected with HIV.

Most probably, the penetration of the virus into the cell is initiated by fusion of the viral and the cellular membrane. In the cytoplasm, a virus coded enzyme, the Reverse Transcriptase (RT,p68,p52) converts the viral single-stranded RNA into a double-stranded DNA. This step is highly specific for the family of retroviruses and contrasts with the usual flow of information in all living cells which goes from DNA to RNA and not vice versa. Next, the viral double-stranded DNA is integrated into the host genome, mediated by the virus coded enzyme

R. P. Baum et al. (eds.), Clinical Use of Antibodies, 169–181.

Table I. Replication cycle of HIV and possibilities for therapeutic interference

	Steps in the replication cycle of HIV	**Therapeutic interference**
1.	Attachment to the cell membrane via the CD4-antigen	Immunization, soluble CD4
2.	Penetration	
3.	Reverse transcription	Inhibition by specific inhibitors (AZT, DDC, DDI, TIBO)
4.	Integration	
5.	Transcription controlled by virus coded proteins	Ribozymes, anti-sense RNA, inhibitors of *tat*, *rev* and other viral regulator proteins
6.	Translation	Ribavirin, interferons?
7.	Particle assembly and budding	Interferons
8.	Maturation (Processing)	Inhibitors of the virus-coded protease

"integrase". From this point of the viral life cycle, the viral genome stays part of the genome of the host cell and behaves there like a cellular gene. For example, if the host undergoes cell division, the viral genetic information will be inherited by both daughter cells.

The expression of viral information is controlled by specific viral genes. The most important roles seem to be played by the genes *tat* and *rev* which are able to shift expression from a latent to a highly active state. For transcription and translation, the cellular machinery is used. The virus particles are assembled just beneath the cell membrane forming buds which are eventually shedded from the cell. Before the particles become infectious they have to undergo a maturation process during which viral precursor proteins are cleaved by a specific viral protease into the final structural proteins as well as the virus coded enzymes. Now, the particles are ready to infect other cells and to start anew the life cycle.

Diagnosis of HIV infection

The most direct way to diagnose an infection is to demonstrate the presence of the infectious agent, and this is also feasible for HIV infection. Usually, the virus is isolated by co-cultivating the sample (e.g.blood) with $CD4^+$ T cell lines or with PBMCs (peripheral blood mononuclear cells, e.g. cord blood cells). However, the procedure is laborious, takes at least a week and does not always, particularly in the early stages of the infection, lead to a positive result. Therefore, virus isolation is not a routine test in HIV diagnostics rather it is mainly used for scientific investigations.

Another possibility is to look for viral antigens with immunological methods. Such test (so called antigen capture assays) are available commercially and are directed towards the detection of the major structural protein of the virus, p24. These tests may be helpful in the diagnosis of the very early phase of the infection where there is a certain degree of viraemia before an antibody response has been mounted. In the later stages, p24 is often not detectable although it reappears during the clinical course and may be used as a prognostic marker during the final stages when its disappearance correlates with the progress of the disease.

Due to the integration of the viral genetic information into the host genome the body has - in contrast to the situation with most of the other virus infections - no chance to clear itself of the virus. This means that the detection of antibodies always indicates an on-going infection while with other viral diseases antibodies are often only signs of earlier infections. Fast and reliable methods for the detection of antibodies are available, and such assays have become the standard procedures for HIV diagnostics.

The technique which allows the most detailed interpretation is the Western Blot assay. In the fist step, a virus preparation is subjected to a SDS polyacrylamide gel electrophoresis (SDS-PAGE) where the viral proteins as well as contaminating proteins are separated according to their size. These proteins are transferred to a membrane without changing their relative position. The membrane is exposed to a serum sample which may contain antibodies able to recognise the respective antigens. This reaction can be visualised with a detection system which leads to a colour deposit on the membrane at the site of the recognised protein. Thus, one can determine whether the antibodies react with contaminating or with viral proteins and, if so, with which viral proteins. Non-specific and specific reactions can be generally easily determined. Criteria have been developed which describe the minimum number of viral proteins and the protein species which have to be recognised by a serum to be scored as positive. This implies that not every reaction with a viral protein indicates an infection. For example, an isolated reaction with p24 is often found with serum of uninfected individuals (Werner et al 1989). The criteria for positivity are now consolidated, and in general, a reaction with at least two of the following viral proteins is scored as positive: p24, gp41 and gp120/160 (Fig.1).

Two general criteria determine the reliability of diagnostic procedures: specificity and sensitivity. They are defined in the following way:

$$\text{Specificity} = \frac{N_x \cdot 100}{N}$$

Nx : No Samples with negative results for test x
N : No samples scored independently negative

$$\text{Sensitivity} = \frac{P_x \cdot 100}{P}$$

P_x : No Samples with positive results for test x
P : No Samples independently scored positive

The basis for these calculations is the definition of groups of individuals which are scored "negative" (N) or "positive (P) by ab independent "absolute" way. In the case of HIV diagnostics, this is mostly done using the Western blot technique as the decisive test. Specificity quantitates the extent of "false positive" results for a given test procedure: the higher the specificity the lower the extent of "false positive" results. In the same way, sensitivity

gure 1. Western Blot

›mmercially available Western Blot stripes ("New LAV Blot I Pasteur") are incubated with selected sera from ·oconversion panels (see Table II). Samples 25 and 26 are identical with samples 2 and 5 from Panel L, nples 27, 28 and 29 with samples 4, 6 and 8 from Panel K and samples 30 and 31 with samples 8 and 15 ım Panel C. Sample 27 is scored as negative as only a faint band with one viral protein (p24) is detectable. In ntrast, sample 28 is positive as, in addition to the p24, the gp160 (the precursor protein for gp120 and gp41) ılso stained. All other sera are clearly positive as they react with different viral proteins.
e sizes of the viral proteins are labelled according to the manufacturer's information.

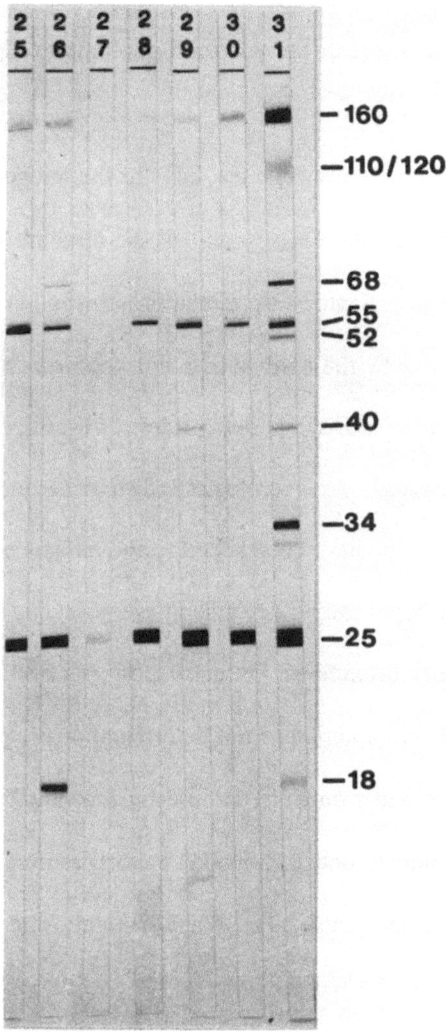

described the extent of "false negative" results.

The test procedures which are most widely used not only for screening large numbers of samples, e.g. blood donations, but also for primary individual diagnosis are based on the principles of the Enzyme Linked Immunosorbent Assay (ELISA). The numerous technical realizations are not within the scope of this contribution. In general, however, viral antigens fixed to a solid support are exposed to the sample. If there are antibodies which recognise the antigen(s) they will stick to the support. After washing away all non-specific antibodies the bound antibodies will be visualized by a detection system which is very similar to that used with Wester blot. The developed dye can be measured photometrically which is a necessary prerequisite for the use in automatic systems.

The main difference between the available test kits are the antigens used. Initially, only whole virus prepared from tissue culture was used. These tests are prone to false positive results as the antigen can be contaminated with cellular proteins and in ELISAs discrimination of which antigens are recognised by the antibodies is not possible. Now there are also kits which use recombinant viral proteins or synthetic peptides. However, even in those tests false positive results have been observed. As a serologically distinct second type of HIV (HIV-2) exists, antigens specific for this type have been added to the antigen mix in some test kits so that infections with both HIV types can be detected in one assay.

All ALISA based test kits licensed in Germany possess sensitivities near 100% and specificities greater than 99%. In addition to the determination of specificity and sensitivity in large groups of blood donors and groups of HIV infected individuals the quality of different test kits is checked by their ability to detect antibodies as early as possible in a panel of serial samples from seroconversion cases (Table 11). What emerged from such studies is that in testing serial samples from an individual case one kit may be superior to another, but with

Table II. Reactivity of different licensed tests in seroconversion follow-up panels*

Test	PEI Reference Serum (Titer)	First bleeding in series scored as positive Panel C	Panel K	Panel L
1	2×10^2	(4)	(4)	(2)
2+	2×10^2	4	6	n.t.
3	5×10^2	n.t.	(4)	2
4	5×10^2	(3)	(4)	n.t.
5+	2×10^3	3	5	1
6	3×10^3	(4)	6	n.t.
7	4×10^3	(5)	6	2
8+	1×10^4	3	5	2
9	6×10^5	(3)	(6)	2

.isted is the first equivocal (in brackets) or positive sample of each serial panel. Early samples in seroconversion panels should ontain low antibody titers. However, the ability of a single test kit to give positive results in early samples is not correlated with s ability to give positive results with higher dilutions of a reference serum.

provided by Boston Biomedica Inc.

Tests containing recombinant or synthetic antigens

.t. not tested

another series the reverse may be true. In conclusion, all licensed test kits are generally sensitive in detecting early seroconversion. However, if there is a strong suspicion of an early HIV infection and if there is a negative test result with one kit, this test should be repeated with another kit which utilizes different antigens. Usually each test procedure is characterised by its own cut off value which seems to form a sharp border between positivity and negativity. In our opinion, the definition of such a cut off value is not sufficient as there are variations in the test procedure. It has to be supplemented by a "grey zone" which stretches from the cut off value into the negative area. Values falling in this grey zone should be interpreted as questionable and have to be confirmed.

How will these types of tests develop in the future? An improvement of sensitivity and specificity seems to be unlikely as both characteristics have reach nearly ideal values. However, the time needed for performing the test could be shorted and the simplicity of the test procedures could be enhanced. Such developments can already be observed. For example, a test kit is available where the results can be read after less than 10 minutes. These kind of tests may be very helpful in emergency situations when a fast diagnosis is essential. However, they may also represent early stages in the design of so called home tests where an individual can perform a diagnostic test with his or her own blood or other body fluid at home without additional help. For a number of reasons, but mainly because of the lack of medical guidance, the German AIDS Council refuses the use of home tests.

Even with the sophisticated ELISA tests which are now available, the possibility of false positive results cannot be excluded. Therefore, a positive test result has to be confirmed before an individual is informed of it. For questionable results where the values fall into the grey zone, the test has to be repeated and if it becomes positive or stays questionable again a confirmatory test has to be performed. The classical confirmatory test, as described earlier, is the Western blot. It may be replaced by immunofluorescence assays if certain conditions are met, i.e. when there is a bright fluorescence with infected cells and no fluorescence at all with uninfected cells.

Last, but not least, it should be mentioned that a new test procedure has emerged, the polymerase chain reaction (PCR). This technique allows the amplification and detection of very tiny amounts of nucleic acids in vitro. It has been already used for diagnosis of HIV infections (ou et al 1988). In theory, by this new method a single piece of nucleic acid in a given sample can be "replicated" by the addition of heat stable DNA polymerase in the presence of two primers. These primers are short oligonucleotides which are needed by the polymerase for its activity and which define the ends of the amplified nucleotide stretch. The "experimental" sensitivity of this assay is very high and approaches or even exceeds that of the direct virus isolation as both methods are based on the replication to detectable levels of the material being looked for. However, this sensitivity is also cause for some concern. The contamination of the test material even with very small amounts of positive samples (e.g. positive controls, see Sarker and Sommer 1990) leads to false positive results. In the early days of diagnostics with PCR, this was the main drawback. In the meantime, devices have been developed which minimize this risk.

PCR was first designed to amplify DNA, and not RNA, which constitutes the genome of many virus families including retroviruses. In this latter case, only the viral genomes already integrated into the host cell genome can be detected directly by PCR. However, the inclusion of reverse transcription by retroviral RT as the first step of PCR opened the possibility to amplify also RNA as DNA. This allows one to look for HIV directly in serum or plasma samples.

The role of PCR in the context of all diagnostic procedure for the detection of HIV infection is not yet absolutely clear. At this time, it is not expected that PCR will replace the established screening procedures, but it will help to find an answer in questionable cases. In addition, it may contribute valuable information o the viral load in the peripheral blood during the course of the disease and during treatment.

Therapy of HIV infection

Due to the ability of the virus to integrate into the host cell genome and to stay there during the whole life span of the infected cell a definite cure must include the elimination or irreversible inactivation of all the integrated viral genomes. Indeed, there are some theoretical concepts on how this goal could be achieved. They include the use of so called ribozymes which recognise and destroy defined sequences of DNA (Sarver et al. 1990). However, all such ideas have still to be substantiated by convincing results of basic research and it is still too early to predict when clinical trials can be expected.

In the meantime, the specific therapy of HIV infection is aimed on the inhibition of the further spread of the virus in an infected individual. The opportunistic infections which are characteristic for AIDS as well as other conditions of the disease demand additional therapeutic support. However, this will not be reviewed in this contribution which has to focus on ways of intervention which are specifically directed on HIV.

Table 1 defines stages in the life of the virus which could be used as targets for therapeutic interference. Of predominant importance is the possibility to inhibit the step which is most characteristic for retroviruses: the reverse transcription. A huge range of compounds able to inhibit reverse transcriptases of animal retroviruses was known and, therefore, soon after the elucidation of the role of HIV in AIDS, a large number of clinical trials with some of these drugs were undertaken. However, so far only one class has turned out to be clinically effective:

the nucleoside analogues. In an extensive study, it could be demonstrated that one of these compounds, azidothymidine AZT (Zidovudine Retrovir ^{TM}) is able to prolong the life span of individuals in late stages of AIDS (Fischl et al.1987). This drug has been licenced since 1987, and it is used extensively. With growing experience, dosage has been reduced and indications have been expanded.

There is no doubt that reverse transcription is very specific for retroviruses. However, it involves a DNA polymerisation step, which is also included in the replication and repair of the cellular genome, performed by cellular DNA polymerases. The question of whether AZT specifically inhibits the viral RT or not could be answered experimentally, and it is clear that although RT is indeed the most sensitive of the known DNA polymerases, at a 10 times higher concentration one of the cellular polymerases (polymerase gamma) is also inhibited (König et al. 1989). This may explain the severe side effects (bone marrow suppression) which is substantial number of treated patients suffer.

Other nucleoside analogues are now under clinical investigation: dideoxycytosine (DDC) and dideoxyinosine (DDI). Unfortunately, they also cause side effects, but these are different from those induced by AZT (DDC: peripheral neurotoxicity, DDI: pancreatitis). These drugs are not yet licenced, but the results available so far may justify attempts at combination therapy where each of the different nucleoside analogues are given at reduced dosage in order to minimize the side effects, but where the inhibiting activity is still ensured.

Recently, very specific inhibitors of HIV-1 RT, which, in contrast to the nucleoside analoga, does not interfere with HIV-2 RT, have been described (Pauwels et al 1990). These belong to a class of benzodiazepin derivatives (TIBO) which until now have not been known to be involved in RT inhibition. It is to be expected that these will be investigated in clinical trials very soon.

All the other therapeutical interventions which are listed in Table 1 have not yet reached clinical significance. However, I expect that one of the different ways to block the adsorption of the virus to the cell could be the subject of a clinical breakthrough prior to other principles which are under investigation. One of the candidates is soluble CD4 which binds to the viral outer membrane protein and thus prevents the interaction between the virus and its cellular receptor, the membrane bound CD4. A similar effect may be exerted by dextran sulfate (Mitsuya et al. 1988) and other polysulfate anions (Biesert et al.1989).

To prevent the virus from entering the cell is also the aim of classical immunization whose benefit in preventing infectious diseases has been demonstrated throughout medical history in many systems. However, there are also concepts which predict a positive influence on the disease by immunization of already infected individuals (Salk 1987). Preliminary studies in monkeys as well as in patients with inactivated complete HIV seem to support this idea (Salk, personal communication). However, the number of the individuals involved is still to small to draw valid conclusions. An extended study is presently under way.

Although not within the scope of this contribution the possibility of preventative immunizations should shortly be discussed. It is already well known that early experiments in animal systems with a wide variety of vaccine candidates failed. However, very recent experiments with inactivated virus as well as with recombinant gp120 (Berman et al.1990) could demonstrate a protective effect. It seems that the first steps in the right direction have now been done. However, there seems to be still a long way to an effective vaccine against HIV due mainly to the problems caused by the variability of the agent.

References

1. Berman P.W. et al (1990) Protection of chimpanzees from infection by HIV-1 after vaccination with recombinant glycoprotein gp120 but not gp160. Nature 345,622-625

2. Biesert L. et al.(1989) Inhibition of HIV and virus replication by polysulphated polyxylan: Hoe/Bay 946, a new antiviral compound. AIDS 2, 449-457

3. Fischl M.A. et al. and Collaborative Working Group (1987) The efficacy of azidothymidine (AZT) in the treatmentof patientswith AIDS and AIDS-relatedcomplex. New.Engl.J.Med. 317,185-191

4. Gelder J. et al. (1990) Potent and selective inhibition of HIV-1 replication in vitro by a novel series of TIBO derivatives Nature 343,470-474

5. König H. et al (1989) Azidothymidine triphosphate is an inhibitor of both human immunodeficiency virus type 1 reverse transcriptase and DNA polymerase gamma.AntimicrobialAgents and Chemotherapy33, 2109-2114

6. Ou C.Y et al.(1988) DNA amplificationfor direct detectionof HIV-1 in DNA of peripheral blood mononuclear cells. Science 239,295-297

7. Salk J.(1987) Prospects for the control of AIDS by immunizing seropositive individuals. Nature 327,473-476

8. Sarker G and Sommer S.S. (1990) Shedding light on PCR contamination. Nature 343,27

9. Sarver N. et al. (1990) Ribozymes as potential anti-HIV-1 therapeutic agents. Science 247,1222-1225

10 Werner A. et al (1989) Antibodies in sera from healthy blood donors and multiple sclerosis patients recognize human and animal retrovirus antigens. Aidsforsch.4,70-73.

INDEX

Developments in Nuclear Medicine

1. P.H. Cox (ed.): *Cholescintigraphy*. 1981 ISBN 90-247-2524-0
2. P.H. Cox (ed.): *Progress in Radiopharmacology*. Selected Topics. Proceedings of the 3rd European Symposium (Noordwijkerhout, The Netherlands, April 1982). 1982 ISBN 90-247-2768-5
3. M.H. Jonckheer and F. Deconinck (eds.): *X-Ray Fluorescent Scanning of the Thyroid*. 1983 ISBN 0-89838-561-X
4. K. Kristensen and E. Nørbygaard (eds.): *Safety and Efficacy of Radiopharmaceuticals*. 1984 ISBN 0-89838-609-8
5. A. Bossuyt and F. Deconinck: *Amplitude/Phase Patterns in Dynamic Scintigraphic Imaging*. With a Foreword by A. Bertrand Brill. 1984 ISBN 0-89838-641-1
6. M.R. Hardeman and Y. Najean (eds.): *Blood Cells in Nuclear Medicine, Part I*. Cell Kinetics and Bio-distribution. 1984 ISBN 0-89838-653-5
7. G.F. Fueger (ed.): *Blood Cells in Nuclear Medicine, Part II*. Migratory Blood Cells. 1984 ISBN 0-89838-654-3
8. H.J. Biersack and P.H. Cox (eds.): *Radioisotope Studies in Cardiology*. 1985 ISBN 0-89838-733-7
9. P.H. Cox, G. Limouris and M.G. Woldring (eds.): *Progress in Radiopharmacology 1985*. 1985 ISBN 0-89838-745-0
10. P.H. Cox, S.J. Mather, C.B. Sampson and C.R. Lazarus (eds.): *Progress in Radiopharmacy*. 1986 ISBN 0-89838-823-6
11. H. Deckart and P.H. Cox (eds.): *Principles of Radiopharmacology*. 1987 ISBN 0-89838-774-4
12. W.-D. Heiss, G. Pawlik, K. Herholz and K. Wienhard (eds.): *Clinical Efficacy of Positron Emission Tomography*. 1987 ISBN 0-89838-898-8
13. G.B. Gerber, H. Métivier and H. Smith (eds.): *Age-related Factors in Radionuclide Metabolism and Dosimetry*. 1987 ISBN 0-89838-953-4
14. K. Kristensen and E. Nørbygaard (eds.): *Safety and Efficacy of Radiopharmaceuticals 1987*. 1987 ISBN 0-89838-986-0
15. C. Beckers, A. Goffinet and A. Bol (eds.): *Positron Emission Tomography in Clinical Research and Clinical Diagnosis*. Tracer Modelling and Radioreceptors. 1989 ISBN 0-7923-0254-0
16. M. De Schrijver: *Scintigraphy of Inflammation with Nanometer-sized Colloidal Tracers*. 1989 ISBN 0-7923-0272-9
17. Ch. Kessler, M.R. Hardeman, H. Henningsen and J.-N. Petrovici (eds.): *Clinical Application of Radiolabelled Platelets*. 1990 ISBN 0-7923-0729-1
18. H.J. Biersack and P.H. Cox (eds.): *Nuclear Medicine in Gastroenterology*. 1991 ISBN 0-7923-1074-8
19. R.P. Baum, P.H. Cox, G. Hör and G.L. Buraggi (eds.): *Clinical Use of Antibodies*. Tumours, infection, infarction, rejection and in the diagnosis of AIDS. 1991 ISBN 0-7923-1424-7

Kluwer Academic Publishers - Dordrecht / Boston / London

MIX
Papier aus verantwortungsvollen Quellen
Paper from responsible sources
FSC® C105338

If you have any concerns about our products,
you can contact us on
ProductSafety@springernature.com

In case Publisher is established outside the EU,
the EU authorized representative is:
Springer Nature Customer Service Center GmbH
Europaplatz 3, 69115 Heidelberg, Germany

Printed by Libri Plureos GmbH
in Hamburg, Germany